GUIDELINES
FOR
EXERCISE TESTING
AND
PRESCRIPTION

Guidelines for Exercise Testing and Prescription has been written by the Preventive and Rehabilitative Exercise Committee of the American College of Sports Medicine. Many individuals on the committee and others from the College have contributed to each edition. The primary responsibility for writing and editing each edition was assumed by the following editorial committees.

First Edition:
- Karl G. Stoedefalke, Ph.D., Co-Chair
- John A. Faulkner, Ph.D., Co-Chair
- Samuel M. Fox, M.D.
- Henry S. Miller, Jr., M.D.
- Bruno Balke, M.D.

Second Edition:
- R. Anne Abbott, Ph.D., Chair
- Karl G. Stoedefalke, Ph.D.
- N. Blythe Runsdorf, Ph.D.
- John A. Faulkner, Ph.D.

Third Edition:
- Steven N. Blair, P.E.D., Chair
- Larry W. Gibbons, M.D.
- Patricia Painter, Ph.D.
- Russell R. Pate, Ph.D.
- C. Barr Taylor, M.D.
- Josephine Will, M.S.

GUIDELINES FOR EXERCISE TESTING AND PRESCRIPTION

AMERICAN COLLEGE OF SPORTS MEDICINE

3rd Edition

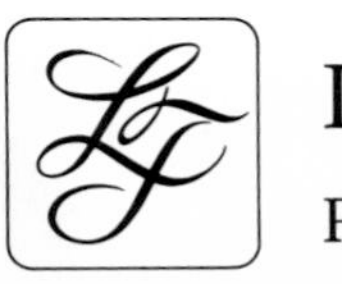

Lea & Febiger

Philadelphia

Lea & Febiger
600 Washington Square
Philadelphia, PA 19106-4198
U.S.A.
(215) 922-1330

Library of Congress Cataloging-in-Publication Data

Main entry under title:

Guidelines for exercise testing and prescription.

Rev. ed. of: Guidelines for graded exercise testing and exercise prescription / American College of Sports Medicine. 1975.
Bibliography: p.
1. Exercise therapy. 2. Cardiacs—Rehabilitation. 3. Exercise tests. I. American College of Sports medicine. II. American College of Sports Medicine. Guidelines for graded exercise testing and exercise prescription.
RC684.E9G85 1986 615.8′24 85-24030
ISBN 0-8121-1022-6

1st Edition, 1975—Reprinted 1976
Reprinted 1977
Reprinted 1979
2nd Edition, 1980—Reprinted 1981
Reprinted 1982 (twice)
Reprinted 1984 (twice)
Reprinted 1985
3rd Edition 1986

Printed in the United States of America

Print Number: 5

Preface

The third edition of this book has been extensively revised. Two new chapters have been added. Chapter 5 deals with exercise for special patient populations. This chapter expands the material on exercise for obese individuals, hypertensive individuals, patients with angina, and patients with other special conditions. Chapter 6 presents principles of behavioral medicine useful in helping clients initiate and maintain a healthy lifestyle. Chapter 2 incorporates the changes in exercise testing that have occurred in recent years. Classification of patients for testing has been simplified, and a section on submaximal testing has been added. Chapter 4 has been extensively revised. Notable changes include expanded sections on cardiac medications and pacemakers. Appendix D, on metabolic calculations, has been completely rewritten. Tables on the energy cost of activities have been moved to Appendix D, so that all information on energy cost is in one place.

The behavioral objectives for all certification tracts have been updated. Two areas of the knowledge base which have been significantly expanded include exercise testing and prescription for pulmonary disease patients, and inpatient exercise programs.

The American College of Sports Medicine has added two new certification programs since the second edition of the *Guidelines.* These new programs, health fitness instructor and health fitness director, reflect the tremendous growth in preventive exercise programs. Additional preventive exercise certification programs are being developed by the American College of Sports Medicine in response to the needs of hundreds of individuals who have a high level of professional training and who apply scientific principles of exercise training and health behavioral change in a variety of community settings. Please contact the College for more information on these new certification programs.

Like the previous editions, many individual clinicians and scientists have contributed to this edition. The American College of Sports Medicine thanks them for their efforts. The College hopes that this third edition of the *Guidelines* will continue to be helpful to practitioners. The ultimate goal is to provide a useful tool which will enhance the quality of programs for our patients, subjects, and participants.

Contents

1

Guidelines for Evaluation of Health Status Prior to Exercise Testing and Prescription

Exercise is a safe activity for most individuals. However, it is desirable for adults to have some screening prior to starting an exercise program or taking an exercise test. It has become apparent that for many individuals the pre-exercise evaluation can be done by non-medical personnel in non-medical settings. Age, health status, type of test, and exercise plan are factors which determine the depth of evaluation required and need for medical involvement. This chapter will focus on the situation when the more comprehensive medical evaluation is appropriate.

A careful evaluation of individuals prior to exercise testing is important for numerous reasons including the following: to assure the safety of exercise testing and subsequent exercise programs, to decide on the appropriate type of exercise test, to identify those in need of more comprehensive medical evaluation, and to prescribe the appropriate type of exercise program following the exercise testing. This evaluation of individuals prior to testing is an integral part of the exercise test protocol.

In general, exercise testing is done for one of the following reasons:

1. To aid in the diagnosis of coronary heart disease in asymptomatic or symptomatic individuals.
2. To assess the safety of exercise prior to starting an exercise program.
3. To assess the cardiopulmonary functional capacity of apparently healthy or diseased individuals.

4. To follow the progress of known coronary or pulmonary disease.
5. To assess the efficacy of various medical and surgical procedures including the effect of medications.

The medical evaluation prior to exercise testing may vary to some extent according to which of these purposes applies.

There are three major categories of individuals who may undergo exercise testing:

1. Apparently healthy—those who are apparently healthy and have no major coronary risk factors.
2. Individuals at higher risk—those who have symptoms suggestive of possible coronary disease and/or at least one major coronary risk factor (Table 1–1).
3. Individuals with disease—those with known cardiac, pulmonary, or metabolic disease.

Results of exercise testing may dictate reclassification of individuals prior to prescribing an exercise program.

APPARENTLY HEALTHY INDIVIDUALS

Apparently healthy individuals under age 45 can usually begin exercise programs without the need for exercise testing as long as the exercise program begins and proceeds gradually and as long as the individual is alert to the development of unusual signs or symptoms. At or above age 45, it is desirable for these individuals to have a maximal exercise test before beginning exercise programs. It is also desirable in those who are already exercising once they reach age 45. A submaximal test is less satisfactory, but useful in some circumstances. At any age, the information gathered from such an exercise test is important to establish an effective and safe exercise prescription. Maximal testing done for individuals at age 35 or above

Table 1–1. Major Coronary Risk Factors

1. History of high blood pressure (above 145/95).
2. Elevated total cholesterol/high density lipoprotein cholesterol ratio (above 5).
3. Cigarette smoking.
4. Abnormal resting ECG—including evidence of old myocardial infarction, left ventricular hypertrophy, ischemia, conduction defects, dysrhythmias.
5. Family history of coronary or other atherosclerotic disease prior to age 50.
6. Diabetes mellitus.

with no symptoms or risk factors should be done under physician supervision. Submaximal testing in apparently healthy individuals of any age can be done without physician attendance, if the testing is carried out by well-trained individuals who are experienced in monitoring exercise tests and in handling emergencies.

INDIVIDUALS AT HIGHER RISK

Individuals at higher risk are those with at least one major coronary risk factor (Table 1–1) and/or symptoms suggestive of cardiopulmonary or metabolic* disease. An exercise test prior to beginning a vigorous exercise program is desirable for high risk individuals of any age. For those without symptoms, an exercise test may not be necessary below age 35 if exercise is undertaken gradually with appropriate guidance and no competitive participation. If maximal exercise tests are done under these circumstances, a physician should be present. Submaximal exercise tests are of little diagnostic use in this population, but if such tests are done, it is not necessary to have a physician present if the patient is under 35 with no symptoms. Persons with symptoms suggestive of coronary, pulmonary or metabolic disease should have a physician supervised maximum exercise test prior to beginning a vigorous exercise program at any age.

PATIENTS WITH DISEASE

Individuals at any age with known cardiovascular, pulmonary, or metabolic disease should have an exercise test prior to beginning vigorous exercise. This is important not only to assess the safety of vigorous exercise, but to measure functional capacity so that progress can be monitored. Exercise testing in this group of individuals is valuable in establishing prognosis and making decisions about need for further evaluation or intervention. A physician should be present.

EVALUATION PRIOR TO TESTING

The depth of evaluation prior to testing will depend on which category of individual (apparently healthy, higher risk, or with disease present) is being tested. In general, however, there are

*Metabolic disease includes diabetes, thyroid disorders, renal disease, liver disease and other less common diseases of a metabolic type.

three major components of the evaluation prior to exercise testing: medical history, physical examination, and laboratory tests.

MEDICAL HISTORY

This is the most important part of the evaluation. Individuals should be questioned about a history of the following:

A. Heart attack, coronary bypass, or other cardiac surgery
B. Chest discomfort—especially with exertion
C. High blood pressure
D. Extra, skipped, or rapid heart beats/palpitations
E. Heart murmurs, clicks, or unusual cardiac findings
F. Rheumatic fever
G. Ankle swelling
H. Peripheral vascular disease
I. Phlebitis, emboli
J. Unusual shortness of breath
K. Lightheadedness or fainting
L. Pulmonary disease including asthma, emphysema and bronchitis
M. Abnormal blood lipids
N. Diabetes
O. Stroke
P. Emotional disorders
Q. Medications of all types
R. Recent illness, hospitalization or surgical procedure
S. Drug allergies
T. Orthopedic problems, arthritis
U. Family* history should be explored for the following:
   1. Coronary disease—at what age
   2. Sudden death—at what age
   3. Congenital heart disease
V. Other habits
   1. Caffeine including cola drinks
   2. Alcohol
   3. Tobacco
   4. Other unusual habits or dieting
   5. Exercise history with information on habitual level of activity: type of exercise, frequency, duration, and intensity.

*Family means grandparents, parents, aunts, uncles and siblings.

PHYSICAL EXAMINATION

A limited physical examination is useful to specifically assess:

A. Weight/body composition
B. Orthopedic problems including arthritis
C. Presence of any acute illness
D. Most significant non-cardiac problems which might influence exercise testing and prescription will be identified through the medical history. Areas of possible concern revealed by the history should be evaluated in the physical examination.
E. Cardiovascular evaluation: The following is an adequate cardiac evaluation prior to exercise testing. If a physician is present this cardiovascular evaluation can easily be carried out in minutes. If the evaluation is being conducted when physician presence is not required, then as much of the evaluation as can be carried out competently should be performed.
    1. Pulse rate and regularity
    2. Blood pressure: supine, sitting, and standing
    3. Auscultation of the lungs with specific attention to:
        a. rales, wheezes, and rhonchi
        b. uniformity of breath sounds in all areas
    4. Palpation for carotid, femoral, and pedal pulses and for cardiac impulse and thrills.
    5. Auscultation of the heart with specific attention to murmurs, gallops, clicks, and rubs
    6. Carotid, abdominal, or femoral bruits
    7. Edema
    8. Xanthoma and xanthelasma

LABORATORY TESTS

Laboratory data are important in the determination of whether an individual fits in the higher risk category. Some laboratory data are helpful prior to testing those with known cardiac, pulmonary, or metabolic disease. The following tests are useful in assessing risk and in assigning individuals to the categories described.

A. Apparently healthy or higher risk individuals
    1. Total cholesterol/high density lipoprotein cholesterol ratio

    2. Triglycerides
    3. Blood glucose
B. Coronary disease
    1. Above tests plus results of all pertinent previous cardiovascular laboratory tests (i.e. angiography, radionuclide studies, previous exercise tests)
    2. Chest x ray
C. Pulmonary disease
    1. Chest x ray
    2. Routine spirometry to include vital capacity and forced expiratory flow volumes
    3. Results of other specialized pulmonary studies

An exercise test can only be interpreted properly with a background of knowledge concerning the individual being tested. The information above is helpful in assuring the safety of the procedure and interpreting the information which is obtained during testing.

Some physicians in private practice find that screening patients prior to increasing habitual exercise is of great value in primary prevention and developing and maintaining patient rapport. Other physicians, because of a lack of facilities or qualified personnel, experience difficulty with exercise screening and exercise prescription. Under these circumstances, a central referral laboratory with qualified technical and medical personnel for exercise testing, prescription, and program supervision may be utilized. The information obtained from the evaluation and testing should be sent promptly to the referring physician and others involved with patient care. This is particulary important for patients who may need immediate medical guidance.

In summary, the limited availability of qualified health personnel and facilities in relation to the large volume of medical evaluations and exercise testing required to comply with the recommendations presented in this chapter (Table 1–2) necessitates discretion in their implementation. The degree of medical supervision of exercise tests proposed varies from situations in which there may be no physician present, to those in which the physician is present but not in visual contact, or times when the physician is in visual contact with the participant. The appropriate protocol is based on the age, health status, and physical activity level of the person to be tested. All

Table 1–2. Guidelines for Exercise Testing

	APPARENTLY HEALTHY		*HIGHER RISK*			*WITH DISEASE*
	Below 45	*45 and Above*	*Below 35 No Symptoms*	*35 and Above No Symptoms*	*Symptoms*	*Any Age*
Maximal Exercise Test Recommended Prior to an Exercise Program	No	Yes	No	Yes	Yes	Yes
Physician Attendance Recommended for Maximal Testing	No (under 35)	Yes	Yes	Yes	Yes	Yes
Physician Attendance Recommended for Sub-maximal Testing	No	No	No	Yes	Yes	Yes

tests should be administered by a person qualified in exercise testing, preferably a person certified as a preventive and rehabilitative exercise test technologist, exercise specialist, or exercise program director or a physician when necessary.

REFERENCES*

Exercise Testing and Training of Apparently Healthy Individuals: A Handbook for Physicians. Dallas, American Heart Association. 1972.

Exercise Testing and Training of Individuals with Heart Disease or at High Risk for its Development: A Handbook for Physicians. Dallas, American Heart Associations. 1975.

American Heart Association. Optimal resources for primary prevention of atherosclerotic diseases. *Circulation, 70,* July 1984.

Ellestad, MH.: *Stress Testing—Principles and Practice.* Philadelphia, F.A. Davis Co., 1982, 2nd edition.

Froelicher, VF.: *Exercise Testing & Training.* New York, LeJacq Publishing Co., 1983.

*These references are also applicable to Chapter 2.

2

Guidelines for Exercise Test Administration

This chapter includes a discussion of the proper procedures and principles of exercise testing in order to insure the reliability of the information obtained and the safety of the person being tested. The guidelines set forth present a rational approach to exercise testing on the premise that qualified personnel may have legitimate reasons for making modifications under specific sets of circumstances.

FIELD TESTING

A field test may be a practical means of exercise testing in some populations, for example where large numbers of apparently healthy individuals such as school children are to be tested. One widely used field test is the 12-minute walk/run test on a measured course. Individuals are instructed to cover the greatest possible distance on the course in a 12-minute period. The distance covered correlates well with maximal oxygen consumption, if the subjects give a maximal effort. Other field tests which use slightly different protocols may also be practical. A home fitness test has been used widely in Canada. The Physical Activity Readiness Questionnaire (PAR-Q) shown in Table 2–1 may be used as a screening method to clear individuals for participating in exercise programs or in an exercise test. Individuals who check yes to any of the PAR-Q questions should not exercise or take an exercise test without further medical clearance. Experience in Canada has shown that the PAR-Q will identify almost all individuals for whom it might be dangerous to start a moderate exercise program or take a submaximal exercise test. After excluding those who do not pass the PAR-Q, individuals step up and down 8-inch steps at an

Table 2–1. Physical Activity Readiness Questionnaire*

For most people, physical activity should not pose any problem or hazard. PAR-Q has been designed to identify the small number of adults for whom physical activity might be inappropriate or those who should have medical advice concerning the type of activity most suitable for them.

1. Has your doctor ever said you have heart trouble?
2. Do you frequently suffer from pains in your chest?
3. Do you often feel faint or have spells of severe dizziness?
4. Has a doctor ever told you that you have a bone or joint problem such as arthritis that has been aggravated by exercise, or might be made worse with exercise?
5. Is there a good physical reason not mentioned here why you should not follow an activity program even if you wanted to?
6. Are you over age 65 and not accustomed to vigorous exercise?

If a person answers yes to any question, vigorous exercise or exercise testing should be postponed. Medical clearance may be necessary.

*Reference: PAR-Q Validation Report,
British Columbia Department of Health
June 1975 (Modified Version).

age and sex specific cadence set by a phonograph record. Fitness is assessed from a combination of test duration and pulse rate after the exercise. This home fitness test has been used safely in large numbers of people.

EXERCISE TEST MODALITIES

Theoretically, exercise tests could be carried out with any form of exercise. Early exercise tests were done by having an individual walk up and down steps at a specified rate for a prescribed duration after which an electrocardiogram (ECG) was taken. The Masters step test is still used in some circumstances, but has largely been eclipsed by newer and more appropriate methods.

The two major modes of exercise testing today are stationary cycling and treadmill walking. In addition, testing with an arm ergometer may be done, but its usefulness is greatest in specific populations. Cycle ergometer tests provide for stable ECG and blood pressure recording. However, individuals who are not accustomed to cycling will often be unable to reach maximal heart rates due to leg fatigue. The rate of cycling is controlled by the patient and not the ergometer, and this may provide a less precise control of work than the treadmill, at least for ergometers with rate dependent exercise intensity.

Treadmill testing is the most common mode of testing because of its wide adaptability. Both speed and elevation can be varied over a wide range of exercise intensities with excellent reproducibility. Walking and even running are natural activities for the vast majority of the population, and it is easy to approach or achieve maximal oxygen consumption and maximal heart rates in individuals who are not limited by musculoskeletal or cardiopulmonary disease. It may be more difficult to obtain exact recordings of the blood pressure and ECG at near maximal work loads with the treadmill. In most circumstances, however, satisfactory recordings can be obtained. Subjects should not be allowed to grasp the railings after the initial stages of testing since this falsely increases the estimated exercise capacity.

Arm testing with an arm crank ergometer is useful in selected patients. Individuals who have lost the use of their legs or have orthopedic or circulatory problems in the lower extremities which limit their ability to do cycle or treadmill exercise can and should be tested with an arm ergometer. Blood pressure can be taken in one arm while the patient continues to crank with the other arm. In addition, in those individuals whose occupational or leisure activity requires sustained upper body effort, arm exercise testing provides useful clinical data. $\dot{V}O_2$ max determined by arm ergometry is less than $\dot{V}O_2$ in leg ergometry and the highest heart rates achieved with arm exercise are usually 10 to 15 beats per minute lower than those achieved with leg exercise.

GENERAL PRINCIPLES OF EXERCISE TESTING

No matter what type of equipment is used, the following principles apply to all exercise testing:

1. The exercise test should begin at a level of intensity considerably below the anticipated limitation or maximal capacity.
2. The exercise intensity should be increased gradually in stages, with observations made at each different stage. The increases in intensity at each stage may be as large as two METs* or more in healthy populations or as small as 1/2 MET in those with disease.
3. Contraindications for testing and indications for stopping exercise should be closely observed.

---

*1 MET = 3.5 ml $O_2 \cdot kg^{-1} \cdot min^{-1}$

4. If in any doubt as to the benefit of testing or the safety of testing, the test should not be performed at that time.
5. Heart rate, blood pressure, patient appearance, rating of perceived exertion (RPE), and patient symptoms (either observed or verbally reported) should be monitored regularly. Grading scales for severity of angina in cardiac patients (Table 2–2) and dypsnea (Table 2–3) in pulmonary patients are especially valuable.
6. All observations should be continued for a 7- to 10-minute recovery unless abnormal responses occur which would require a longer post-test observation.
7. Exercise tolerance in METs should be calculated from the treadmill or ergometer protocol used, or measured directly if oxygen uptake is obtained.
8. The testing area should be 22° C (72° F) or less and the humidity 60% or less if possible.

INFORMED CONSENT

Individuals should sign an informed consent form prior to exercise testing. A sample consent form is included in Appendix A. The purpose of the consent form is to make certain the patient is aware of the small, but real risk of exercise testing. This risk, according to present data, is approximately one death (and three cardiac events*) per 10,000 tests in large, varied populations. More important than having a patient sign a consent form is taking the time to explain possible risks, the pur-

Table 2–2. Angina Scale

1+	Light, barely noticeable
2+	Moderate, bothersome
3+	Severe, very uncomfortable
4+	Most severe pain ever experienced in the past

Table 2–3. Dyspnea Scale

1.	Mild-noticeable to patient—not to observer
2.	Some difficulty—noticeable to observer
3.	Moderate difficulty—but can continue
4.	Severe difficulty—patient cannot continue

*A cardiac event is a serious arrhythmia or heart attack.

pose of testing, and the testing protocol itself. Clear and complete instructions prior to testing will significantly reduce patient anxiety. It is important to give patients time to ask questions prior to testing. Even though the verbal explanation of risks is more important than the signed consent, it is still necessary that the signed consent form be completed as a written piece of evidence that the verbal conversation did take place. The consent form should include a statement that the patient has been given an opportunity to ask questions about the procedure and has sufficient information to give the informed consent. If the subject to be tested is a minor, a legal guardian or parent must sign the consent form.

CONTRAINDICATIONS TO TESTING

There are certain individuals for whom the risks of testing outweigh the potential benefits. These individuals should not be tested. There are other individuals whose medical conditions increase the risk of testing. It is important in these circumstances for the test administrator to weigh carefully the anticipated benefits and determine that these outweigh the risks. Table 2–4 and 2–5 outline contraindications and relative contraindications for exercise testing. Some of these points do not apply in the circumstances where an individual is being tested for specific reasons after a myocardial infarction or surgical procedure. Guidelines for testing in these special circumstances are outlined in a subsequent section.

For an initial diagnostic exercise test, it is often helpful to

Table 2–4. Contraindications to Exercise Testing

1. Recent acute myocardial infarction
2. Unstable angina
3. Uncontrolled ventricular dysrhythmia
4. Uncontrolled atrial dysrhythmia which compromises cardiac function
5. Congestive heart failure
6. Severe aortic stenosis
7. Suspected or known dissecting aneurysm
8. Active or suspected myocarditis
9. Thrombophlebitis or intracardiac thrombi
10. Recent systemic or pulmonary embolus
11. Acute infection
12. Third degree heart block
13. Significant emotional distress (psychosis)
14. A recent significant change in the resting ECG
15. Acute pericarditis

Table 2–5. Relative Contraindications to Exercise Testing

1. Resting diastolic blood pressure over 120 mm Hg or resting systolic blood pressure over 200 mm Hg
2. Moderate valvular heart disease
3. Digitalis or other drug effect
4. Electrolyte abnormalities
5. Fixed rate artificial pacemaker
6. Frequent or complex ventricular irritability
7. Ventricular aneurysm
8. Cardiomyopathy including hypertrophic cardiomyopathy
9. Uncontrolled metabolic disease (diabetes, thyrotoxicosis, myxedema, etc.)
10. Any serious systemic disorder (mononucleosis, hepatitis, etc.)
11. Neuromuscular, musculoskeletal, or rheumatoid disorders which would make exercise difficult

have the patient off all medication if there are no adverse effects from doing so and if the referring physician agrees. As a rule it is helpful to have patients on recommended medications for follow-up evaluations so that response to medication can be evaluated.

PATIENT INSTRUCTIONS

Patients should abstain from food, tobacco, alcohol, and caffeine for at least 3 hours prior to testing. If possible, it is helpful for patients to avoid alcohol, caffeine, and tobacco for longer periods of time prior to testing. Women should bring a loose fitting blouse that buttons down the front with short sleeves and should avoid restrictive undergarments such as panty hose or a girdle. It is best to wear a snug fitting bra made of something other than nylon. Clothing should permit freedom of movement and include a comfortable walking/running shoe.

PREPARATION FOR TESTING

Electrode sites should be rubbed with alcohol to remove skin oils and rubbed with a mild abrasive agent, such as a scouring pad, until the skin is erythematous. This removes the superficial layer of skin. Proper skin preparation will produce some patient discomfort. An electrolyte cream or gel is applied for conduction (unless already present on disposable electrodes), and the electrode is placed on the skin. It is best, if possible, to avoid placing the electrode over large muscle masses. It is not necessary to shave electrode sites for most electrodes.

LEADS

Many different lead systems have been used for exercise testing. Single lead systems may be adequate in young, healthy populations where the primary purpose of testing is to measure fitness. However, it is much preferred to use as many leads as is practical. In higher risk or diseased populations, it is essential to use at least 1 lead which looks at the inferior wall of the heart (i.e. lead II), 1 lead which looks at the anterior wall of the heart (i.e. VI), and 1 which lies over the lateral precardial area (i.e. lead V5). The Frank lead system covers these three important areas, but a 12-lead system is usually preferred. Significant loss of sensitivity may result if only 1 or 2 leads are used for monitoring subjects.

ECG RECORDINGS

A standard resting ECG must be obtained prior to beginning a test. The ECG should be constantly observed on an oscilloscope during testing. Standard ECG strips should be recorded at 1- to 5-minute intervals or at a minimum during each stage during testing. If questionable abnormalities appear, readings may be taken at more frequent intervals. It is helpful to have a delay switch so that premature beats or dysrhythmias which may occur can be recorded or documented. When the test is terminated, it is useful to have a brief (1 to 3 minutes) cool down at a lower exercise intensity before stopping the test, in order to minimize the risk of hypotension from venous pooling. Immediately after this cool down, patients should be supine to increase the sensitivity of exercise testing. The supine position increases venous return and may be more likely to produce diagnostic ECG abnormalities. Monitoring should continue for approximately 10 minutes during recovery or longer if abnormalities are still present. Some tests may be abnormal only in the recovery period and not during exercise.

BLOOD PRESSURE RECORDING

Blood pressure should be taken in the supine, sitting, and standing positions prior to exercise. Thereafter, blood pressures should be monitored every 2 to 5 minutes or at each stage of the test. Blood pressure should be measured more often in the presence of hypo- or hypertensive readings. During recovery, blood pressure is usually monitored at 2- to 3-minute intervals.

Blood pressure should be measured with the subject's arm relaxed and not grasping a treadmill bar or cycle handle bar. The use of an appropriate sized blood pressure cuff is important to insure accurate readings.

MAXIMAL VS. SUBMAXIMAL TESTING

A maximal exercise test brings an individual to a level of intensity where fatigue or symptoms prohibit further exercise or when maximal oxygen consumption* ($\dot{V}O_2$ max) is achieved and no further increase in heart rate occurs. Estimates of predicted maximal heart rate may be used as a guide for test termination, but these estimates should not be used as predetermined termination points in maximal testing. The range of maximal heart rates at any age is large, even for apparently healthy adults. A submaximal exercise test takes the subject to a predetermined endpoint. This predetermined endpoint can be 85% of predicted maximal heart rate, achievement of a predetermined exercise intensity, or achievement of a certain level on a perceived exertion scale.

Submaximal testing may be useful for determination of fitness where a diagnostic test is not required, i.e. in apparently healthy individuals. $\dot{V}O_2$ max can be predicted from submaximal tests, however the results are often unreliable. A target heart rate set arbitrarily may be close to or at maximal for some individuals and far below maximal for other individuals. Submaximal exercise tests may have some value in predicting risk of coronary disease in the asymptomatic patient. However, a significant degree of coronary insufficiency is generally required to produce an abnormal ECG response, and the submaximal test is less likely to bring the patient to a level of intensity that will produce meaningful ECG or blood pressure changes.

At any given submaximal exercise level, a trained individual will have a lower heart rate than the untrained individual of the same age and sex. As an individual becomes more fit, the heart rate decreases at a given submaximal intensity. Thus, submaximal testing may be useful in monitoring changes in fitness resulting from an exercise program through the comparison of heart rates obtained during submaximal exercise. The following

---

*Greatest rate of oxygen uptake observed during exercise; indicated by failure of oxygen uptake to increase with increase in external work.

section outlines a simple ergometer test which has been developed for field use in a community health survey and has been used safely in testing large numbers of individuals without physician supervision. More than 30,000 of these tests have been administered in a worksite health promotion program with no mortality or serious morbidity.

SUBMAXIMAL CYCLE ERGOMETER EXERCISE TEST (EXAMPLE)

Cycle ergometry is a non-weight bearing activity and larger individuals with greater muscle mass will have a performance advantage. Therefore, modifications must be made into account the patient's weight. One of three protocols (Table 2–6) is selected according to the subject's weight and activity status as outlined in Table 2–7. Activity status is subjectively determined by the test administrator from reviewing questionnaire data provided by the participant or by verbal query. Individuals who have been regularly participating (the last 3 months) in vigorous activities for at least 15 minutes, 3 times per week, are classified as very active.

Exercise heart rates are monitored during the test by palpation of the pulse or by electronic monitoring. Heart rate is checked during the last 15 seconds of each test stage, and the test is terminated when the heart rate reaches 65 to 70% of the predicted age-adjusted maximal heart rate (Table 2–8). These per-

Table 2–6. Test Protocols

	Test Stages (minutes)			
Protocol	*I (1–2)*	*II (3–4)*	*III (5–6)*	*IV (7–8)*
A	*25 (150)	50 (300)	75 (450)	100 (600)
B	25 (150)	50 (300)	100 (600)	150 (900)
C	50 (300)	100 (600)	150 (900)	200 (1200)

*Workload in watts (kilogram meters per minute)

Table 2–7. Protocol Selection Criteria

Body Weight in kg (lbs)	*Very Active*	
	No	*Yes*
<73 (160)	A	A
74–90 (161–199)	A	B
>91 (200)	B	C

Table 2–8. Target Heart Rate for Cycle Ergometer

Age (years)	*Heart Rate (beats/minute)*
<20	140
20–29	135
30–39	130
40–49	120
50–59	115
60–65	110

centages of maximal heart rate will be inaccurate in individuals who are taking drugs which blunt the heart rate response to exercise.

Heart rate is measured for at least two and preferably three test stages. A rough estimate of $\dot{V}O_2$ max can then be extrapolated using the predicted age-adjusted maximal heart as illustrated in Figure 2–1.

MAXIMAL EXERCISE TESTING

The remaining guidelines in this chapter deal primarily with maximal testing though some of the principles outlined are applicable to submaximal testing as well. Maximal exercise testing has advantages over submaximal testing in most circumstances.

TEST PROTOCOLS

A number of different treadmill and cycle ergometer protocols are widely used. Figure 2–2 presents four of the most common treadmill protocols.

MAXIMAL CYCLE ERGOMETER PROTOCOL (EXAMPLE)

Cycle ergometer exercise protocols may be adapted to fit the needs of the subject being tested just as different treadmill protocols are chosen or standard protocols modified.

1. Adjust height of the saddle and handle bar to fit the patient. The knees should be flexed at approximately 5° when the foot is at its lowest point. Subject should be instructed not to grip the handlebars tightly.
2. Pedal speed should be constant throughout at 50 to 60 rpm.
3. Begin the test by having the subject pedal with the lowest resistance possible on the bike for a 2-minute warmup.
4. Increase external work by 25 to 50 watts (150 to 300 kg)

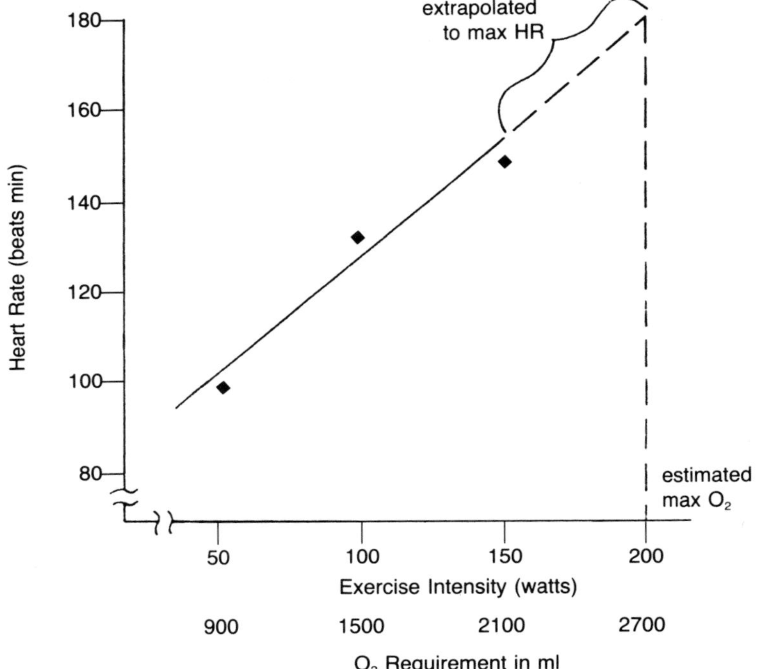

FIGURE 2–1. Heart rate obtained from at least three submaximal exercise intensities may be extropolated to the age predicted maximal heart rate. A vertical line to the intensity scale estimates maximal exercise intensity. (Adapted from: Blair SN.: *Behavioral Health: A Handbook of Health Enhancement and Disease Prevention.* Matarazzo JD, et al. (eds). New York, John Wiley & Sons, 1984, p. 438).

per stage. The increase in intensity depends on weight and fitness of the subject. The duration of each stage should be 2 to 3 minutes.

5. The heart rate should be taken every 1 to 2 minutes and the blood pressure measured during the last minute of the stage with the arm free from gripping the handlebar.
6. The ECG is recorded at the end of each stage or more frequently if indicated.
7. Termination points are similar to those described for treadmill testing.
8. For recovery, decrease the intensity and continue pedalling for up to 10 minutes. Blood pressure, heart rate and ECG should be monitored throughout recovery.

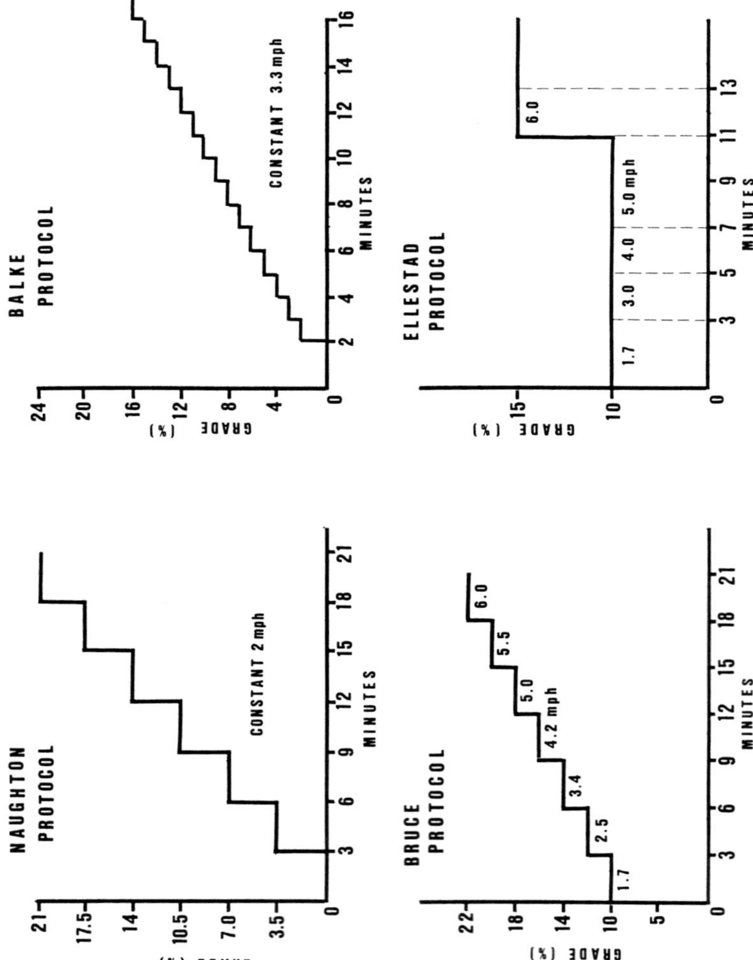

FIGURE 2–2. Four commonly used treadmill protocols are shown in this figure.

OBSERVATION OF TESTING

Ideally, a diagnostic test becomes an extension of the physical examination itself. The physician or other certified professional conducting the test gains the most information by observing the patient prior to, during, and following testing. There is a great deal besides the ECG that should be monitored, including patient appearance, blood pressure, heart rate response, presence or absence of symptoms, and functional capacity. These are as important as the ECG itself. Criteria for stopping a test are listed in Table 2–9. In some settings clinical judgment may indicate continuing a test in the presence of these conditions.

CRITERIA FOR AN ABNORMAL EXERCISE TEST

Table 2–10 lists those occurrences which constitute an abnormal response to exercise testing. These abnormal responses may or may not be a result of ischemia.

ST-elevation generally indicates severe disease or a wall motion abnormality. The combination of ST-depression or elevation and ventricular irritability often indicates multi-vessel coronary disease.

Table 2–9. Indications for Stopping an Exercise Test

1. Subject requests to stop.
2. Failure of the monitoring system.
3. Progressive angina (stop at 3+ level or earlier on a scale of 1+ to 4+) (see Table 2–2).
4. Two millimeters horizontal or downsloping ST-depression or elevation.
5. Sustained supraventricular tachycardia.
6. Ventricular tachycardia.
7. Exercise induced left or right bundle branch block.
8. Any significant drop (10 mm Hg) of systolic blood pressure, or failure of the systolic blood pressure to rise with an increase in exercise load after the initial adjustment period.
9. Lightheadedness, confusion, ataxia, pallor, cyanosis, nausea, or signs of severe peripheral circulatory insufficiency.
10. Excessive blood pressure rise: Systolic greater than 250 mm Hg; diastolic greater than 120 mm Hg.
11. R on T premature ventricular complexes.
12. Unexplained inappropriate bradycardia—pulse rise slower than two standard deviations below age-adjusted normals.
13. Onset of second or third degree heart block.
14. Multifocal PVCs.
15. Increasing ventricular ectopy (see #3 in Table 2–10).

Table 2–10. Criteria for an Abnormal Exercise Test

1. One millimeter or more of exercise induced ST-segment depression or elevation relative to the Q-Q line, lasting .08 seconds or more from the J-point.
2. Chest discomfort typical of angina pectoris induced or increased by exercise.
3. Ventricular tachycardia or frequent (>30%) premature ventricular contractions, or multifocal premature ventricular contractions.
4. Exercise induced left or right bundle branch block.
5. Significant drop (greater than 10 mm Hg) in systolic blood pressure during exercise, or failure of the systolic blood pressure to rise with an increase in exercise intensity after the initial adjustment period.
6. Sustained supraventricular tachycardia.
7. R on T PVCs.
8. Exercise induced second or third degree heart block.
9. Post-exercise U-wave inversion.
10. Inappropriate bradycardia.

LEVEL OF EXERTION

Maximal heart rate varies greatly among individuals during exercise testing. Therefore, it is helpful to be able to evaluate the level of exertion in order to assess whether or not a test is truly maximal and to assess when maximum exercise is being approached. This may be even more essential if patients are taking medication that blunts the heart rate response to exercise. Perceived exertion scales such as those illustrated Figure 2–3 provides a means to quantify subjective exercise intensity. Such subjective estimates of exercise intensity by the person being tested have been found to correlate well (0.80 to 0.90) with oxygen uptake and heart rate. The chart is placed within easy view, and the patient is queried periodically as to the level of perceived exertion. Unless symptoms intervene, exercise is considered to be maximal or near maximal when the patient reports a perceived exertion of 19 or 20 (or 9 to 10 on the new scale).

PULMONARY PATIENTS

In pulmonary patients, initial exercise intensities should be low, and the size of incremental increases should usually be small. In addition to the data mentioned previously, measurements which quantify ventilation, breathing frequency, and tidal volume should be made. These measurements can be obtained by dry gas meter, tissot spirometer, or flow meter. Direct measurement of $\dot{V}O_2$ in pulmonary patients is especially helpful, as are ear oximetry or arterial blood gasses. During testing,

RPE		New Rating Scale	
6		0	Nothing at all
7	Very, very light	0.5	Very, very weak
8		1	Very weak
9	Very light	2	Weak
10		3	Moderate
11	Fairly light	4	Somewhat strong
12		5	Strong
13	Somewhat hard	6	
14		7	Very strong
15	Hard	8	
16		9	
17	Very hard	10	Very, very strong
18			Maximal
19	Very, very hard		
20			

FIGURE 2–3. The original rating of perceived exertion scale and the revised ratio scale may be used in exercise testing or exercise programs. (Reference: Borg GV.: *Med Sci Sports Exercise, 14*:377–87, 1982).

it is helpful to quantify dyspnea during the test and recovery, using a scale such as one in Table 2–3.

The major purpose of exercise testing pulmonary patients is usually to measure functional status. In addition, testing may help differentiate cardiac from pulmonary dypsnea and aid in the prescription of home supplemental oxygen. Maximal heart rates achieved may be lower in pulmonary patients than in cardiac patients. Epinephrine, aminophyllin, (in addition to cardiac emergency drugs) and oxygen should always be on hand when pulmonary patients are being tested.

EARLY POST-INFARCTION OR POST-SURGERY EXERCISE TESTING

It is often useful to test individuals soon after myocardial infarction or surgical procedure, just prior to hospital discharge or a few weeks post-discharge. This type of test can be a valuable indicator of future prognosis and the need for further diagnostic studies or therapy. Patients who manifest abnormalities on exercise testing soon after infarction or surgical procedure are more likely to have complications.

Individuals with normal exercise tests soon after myocardial infarction or surgical procedure are much less likely to have future problems and can often be quickly returned to full occupational and recreational activity.

Pre-discharge or early post-discharge (i.e. 3 weeks) exercise tests are usually submaximal. Prior to testing, patients should be ambulatory and be able to climb one flight of stairs. Drugs should not be withdrawn for testing. A low level exercise test starting with the treadmill flat and a speed of 2 mph with an increase of 1 MET every 2 minutes may be used. A sample predischarge protocol would take patients to 70% of predicted maximal heart rate, 5 METS, angina, a specified level of exertion, or any of the previously outlined reasons for stopping an exercise test, whichever occurs first. Three to 4 weeks after infarction, many patients may be able to tolerate a symptom limited test without predetermined end points, although in many cases there may be no reason to test to that level.

EMERGENCIES

All personnel concerned with exercise testing should be trained in cardiopulmonary resuscitation. Telephone numbers for emergency assistance should be clearly posted on all telephones. Evacuation plans should be established and posted. Regular drills should be conducted at least quarterly for new personnel.

If a problem occurs during exercise testing, the physician available should be immediately summoned if not present. The physician should make the decision whether or not to call for evacuation to the nearest hospital if testing is not carried out in the hospital. If a physician is not available and there is any question as to the status of the patient, then emergency transportation to the closest hospital should be immediately summoned. Except for defibrillation, placing an intravenous catheter, and treatment of ventricular dysrhythmias, advanced cardiac life support should usually be carried out in the hospital and not in the testing station unless the physician present is experienced and competent in all aspects of Advanced Cardiac Life Support. The following equipment should be available in any area where maximal exercise testing is performed in a medical setting.

1. Defibrillator with electrode paste
2. Airway
3. Oxygen
4. Intravenous sets including fluids
5. Intravenous canulas
6. Intravenous stand
7. Syringes and needles in multiple sizes
8. Adhesive tape
9. AMBU bag with pressure release valve
10. Suction equipment

Drugs
1. Aromatic ammonia
2. Metaraminol (Aramine)
3. Furosemide (Lasix)
4. Epinephrine
5. Atropine
6. Isoproterenol (Isuprel)
7. Calcium chloride
8. Sodium bicarbonate
9. Lidocaine
10. Amyl nitrate ampule
11. Digoxin—I.V. and tablets
12. Nitroglycerin tablets
13. Verapamil (Isoptin)
14. I.V. Propranolol (Inderal)
15. I.V. Diazepam (Valium)
16. Dopamine
17. I.V. Nitroglycerin

CALCULATION OF FUNCTIONAL STATUS

Under proper conditions as outlined in these guidelines, the exercise intensity achieved on a standard maximal treadmill or cycle ergometer exercise test is a useful estimate of maximal oxygen consumption unless abnormalities force premature cessation of exercise. The formulas given in Appendix D may be used to calculate the oxygen demand for the exercise intensity achieved during an exercise test. These estimates may be useful in comparing workloads from different test protocols. Figure 2–4 allows estimation of maximal oxygen uptake and exercise capacity in METs from treadmill time or cycle ergometer exercise intensity. Actual measurement of maximal oxygen con-

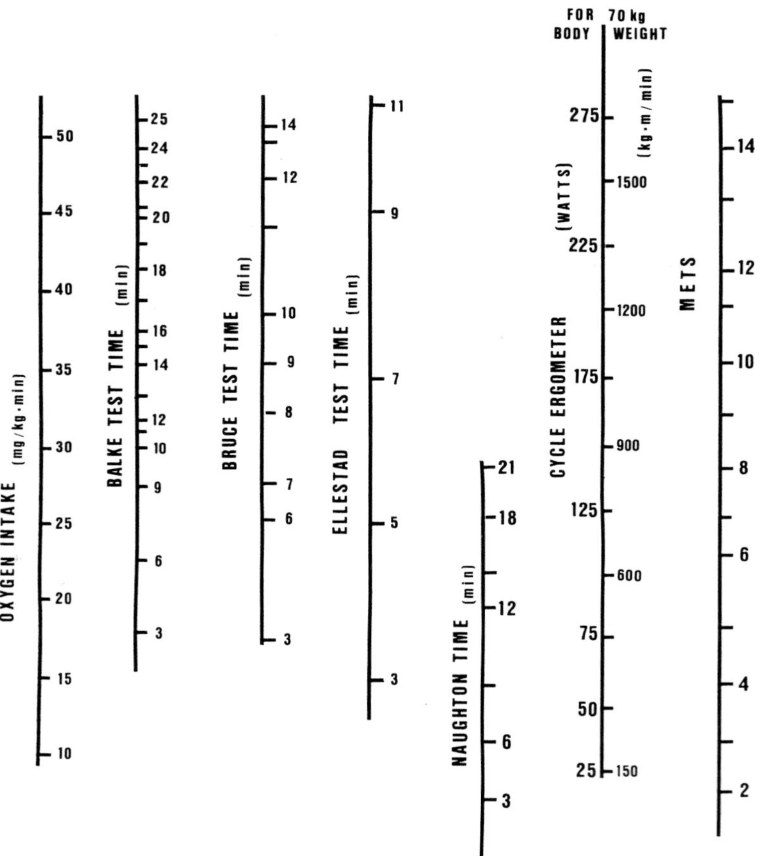

FIGURE 2–4. Exercise intensity equivalents can be estimated by drawing a horizontal line from the time on a given treadmill or cycle ergometer protocol to oxygen uptake (on the left) or MET level (on the right). Modified from: Pollock ML, et al.: *Am Heart J, 92*:39–46, 1976).

sumption may be desirable in certain research laboratory situations, but for testing large numbers of individuals, or in a clinical setting, this is usually impractical. The measurement of $\dot{V}O_2$ max requires appropriate gas analyses equipment, breathing valves, etc.

It should be remembered that follow up exercise tests will often show increased estimated functional capacity even when little if any change has occurred in peak oxygen uptake. This is a result of the learning phenomenon since the patient is acquainted with the procedure on subsequent tests.

INTERPRETATION

It is important to use all available information in the interpretation of an exercise test in the diagnosis of coronary disease as outlined in the section on observation of testing. In addition to information collected during testing on the electrocardiogram, blood pressure, symptoms, RPE, etc., interpreting an exercise test requires knowledge of the risk factors and clinical status of the person being tested. An exercise test cannot be interpreted in a vacuum. No one should be told that they have or do not have coronary disease based on exercise test results alone. False positive and false negative results occur.

FALSE POSITIVE AND FALSE NEGATIVE TESTS

An exercise test interpreted as abnormal in a person who is found not to have disease is called a false positive test. A test interpreted as normal in a person who is found to have disease is called a false negative test. The probability of a false positive test is related to the *specificity* of a test. For example, if 100 people are free of disease and an exercise test is normal in 90 of the 100, then the specificity of the test is 90%. The other 10% are false positives. Where the specificity is high, those without disease will more likely be correctly identified as being disease free, and there will be few false positive tests. On the other hand, false negative test results relate to the *sensitivity* of a test. If for example, there are 100 people with disease, and the test correctly identifies 90 of those people by their having an abnormal test, the sensitivity of the test is 90% and there are 10% false negatives. Where the sensitivity is high, those with disease are correctly identified as having disease, and there will be few false negatives.

Exercise test specificity is reported to be in the range of 80 to 90% for men. Women are reported to have a greater frequency of false positive exercise tests than men, thus the specificity is lower (about 70%). Individuals who have S-T segment abnormalities during hyperventilation may also exhibit false positive exercise tests. For this reason, many laboratories have the subject hyperventilate for 30 seconds prior to the exercise test to evaluate any S-T segment changes.

Sensitivity for exercise testing is reported to be in the range of 60 to 80%. Many studies which reported low sensitivity of exercise testing were not done under optimal circumstances using multiple ECG leads or were not maximal tests. Thus the true sensitivity of exercise testing may be higher than is reported in some studies. Conditions and circumstances in which false positive or false negative tests may occur are listed in Tables 2–11 and 2–12.

The likelihood that an abnormal test represents true coronary disease is directly related to the prevalence of disease in that population. In other words, in populations where the prevalence of disease is low (i.e. young asymptomatic individuals) an abnormal test is much more likely to be a false positive test than is an abnormal test in a population with a high prevalence of disease (i.e. older individuals with coronary risk factors). Thus, an individual's pre-test probability of having coronary disease based on age, sex, risk factors, symptoms, etc. strongly influences how one interprets an abnormal response in that individual. Useful graphs have been developed which give a quantitative estimate of this probability of disease based on

Table 2–11. Causes of False Positive Tests

1. A pre-existing abnormal resting ECG (for example ST-T abnormalities)
2. Cardiac hypertrophy
3. Wolff-Parkinson-White syndrome and other conduction defects
4. Hypertension
5. Drugs (e.g., digitalis)
6. Cardiomyopathy
7. Hypokalemia
8. Vasoregulatory abnormalities
9. Sudden intense exercise
10. Mitral valve prolapse syndrome
11. Pericardial disorders
12. Pectus excavatum
13. Technical or observer error

Table 2–12. Causes of False Negative Tests

1. Failure to reach an adequate exercise workload
2. Insufficient number of leads to detect ECG changes
3. Failure to use other information such as systolic blood pressure drop, symptoms, dysrhythmias, heart rate response, etc., in test interpretation
4. Single vessel disease
5. Good collateral circulation
6. Musculoskeletal limitations before cardiac abnormalities occur
7. Technical or observer error

these pre-test probabilities and the magnitude of ST segment depression or elevation during the test.

The predictive value of an abnormal test is high in groups with a high prevalence of CHD. Conversely, in populations where the prevalence of disease is low, the predictive value of a normal test is high. This latter circumstance is particularly relevant to the "clearance" of persons wishing assurance that latent disease is unlikely.

INTERPRETING ST-SEGMENT DEPRESSION

Persistent ST-segment depression (at least 1 mm that is horizontal or downsloping at .08 seconds after the J point) that occurs early in exercise and remains throughout the test is more likely to be due to coronary disease than ST-depression that occurs only at high exercise intensity. The depth and the slope of ST-segment depression are both important. Horizontal or downsloping ST-depression is more likely a result of coronary insufficiency that upsloping ST-segment depression. Those with 2 or 3 mm of ST-segment depression are more likely to have coronary insufficiency than those with 1 mm of ST-segment depression. Subjects who manifest abnormalities but have excellent functional capacities are less likely to have significant coronary disease than individuals who manifest the same abnormalities but are unfit. Computerized interpretation of exercise tests may enhance the interpretation of questionable tracings. Computerized ECGs may also allow greater reproducibility and make comparison easier between tests done at different times on the same patient or tests done on different patients.

FOLLOW-UP

Most individuals who have abnormal exercise tests at moderate or high levels of exertion do not need to have coronary angiography. Many individuals with abnormal exercise responses can be followed with periodic exercise tests to see if the abnormalities observed increase with time. Patients with an abnormal exercise response who manifest greater abnormality on subsequent tests or the same abnormality at a lower exercise level are more likely to have coronary insufficiency caused by progressive atherosclerosis and may require coronary angiography. Serial testing increases sensitivity.

Non-invasive radionuclide studies may be done to assess further the likelihood that an abnormal exercise test is the manifestation of coronary disease. These tests are especially useful to help interpret abnormal test results in the absence of symptoms or multiple risk factors, and normal test results in subjects with suggestive symptoms.

PATIENT BRIEFING

Patient education following the exercise test is one of the most important, but often neglected, components of exercise testing. If agreeable with the referring physician, it is important to clearly explain to each patient the relevant findings and their significance. Care should be taken not to make an absolute diagnosis on the basis of exercise test results alone. Patients should be told about risks and likelihood of disease rather than presence or absence of disease. This period of discussion and explanation following the test is also a good time to further observe the effect of exercise on the patient. Most complications as a result of exercise testing occur during the recovery period, not during the exercise period itself. Patients should be given information on the ECG, blood pressure response, pulse rate, and fitness level. It is often helpful to have a chart available to show patients their achieved fitness level and how this compares with averages and norms for patients in similar age groups. Discussion of the appropriate exercise heart rate and principles of aerobic exercise may begin at this time.

REFERENCES

Exercise Testing and Training of Apparently Healthy Individuals: A Handbook for Physicians. Dallas, American Heart Association. 1972.

Exercise Testing and Training of Individuals with Heart Disease or at High Risk for its Development: A Handbook for Physicians. Dallas, American Heart Association. 1975.

American Heart Association. Optimal resources for primary prevention of atherosclerotic diseases. *Circulation, 70,* July 1984.

Ellestad, MH.: *Stress Testing—Principles and Practice.* Philadelphia, F.A. Davis Co., 1975.

Froelicher, VF.: *Exercise Testing & Training.* New York, LeJacq Publishing Co., 1983.

Shephard RJ, Bailey DA, Mirwald RL.: Development of the Canadian home fitness test. *Can Med Assn J, 114*:675–682, 1976.

3

Principles of Exercise Prescription

An exercise prescription should designate the type, intensity, duration, frequency and progression of physical activity. These five components are applicable to the development of exercise programs for persons regardless of age, functional capacity and presence or absence of disease states. The maximal safe exercise prescription for any individual is best determined from an objective measurement of physical fitness including observations of heart rate, ECG, arterial blood pressure and functional capacity obtained during an exercise test.

This chapter presents the general principles that should be applied in developing exercise prescriptions to enhance the health related components of physical fitness (i.e., cardiorespiratory endurance, body composition, flexibility and muscular strength and endurance). Subsequent chapters address the specific considerations that pertain to exercise prescription for cardiac patients and other diseased persons.

CARDIORESPIRATORY FITNESS

Based on the existing evidence concerning exercise prescription for asymptomatic adults, the American College of Sports Medicine has made the following recommendations for the quantity and quality of exercise for developing and maintaining cardiorespiratory fitness and body composition (*Med Science Sports Exercise 10*: VII-X, 1978).

• Type of activity: Any activity that uses large muscle groups, that can be maintained for a prolonged period, and is rhythmical and aerobic in nature, e.g. running-jogging, walking-hiking, swimming, skating, bicycling, rowing, cross-country skiing, rope skipping, and various endurance game activities.

• Intensity of conditioning: Physical activity corresponding to 65 to 90% of maximal heart rate or 50 to 85% of $\dot{V}O_2$ max (functional capacity).

• Duration of conditioning: 15 to 60 minutes of continuous or discontinuous aerobic activity. Duration is dependent on the intensity of the activity, thus lower intensity activity should be conducted over a longer period of time. Endurance conditioning is more readily attained in longer duration programs. Lower to moderate intensity activity of longer duration is recommended for non-athletic adults because of potential hazards and compliance problems associated with high intensity activity.

• Frequency of conditioning: 3 to 5 days per week.

• Rate of progression: In most cases, the conditioning effect allows individuals to increase the total work done per session. In continuous exercise this occurs by an increase in intensity, duration, or by some combination of the two. The most significant conditioning effects may be observed during the first 6 to 8 weeks of the exercise program. The physician, exercise program director, exercise specialist, health fitness instructor or health fitness director should adjust the exercise prescription as these conditioning effects occur with the adjustment depending on participant characteristics, new exercise test results or on the exercise performance during exercise sessions.

The principles of exercise prescription are similar for the asymptomatic and the symptomatic participant. The difference arises in the manner in which the principles are applied, i.e., higher intensity vs. lower intensity, longer duration vs. short duration, daily exercise vs. 3 times per week frequency, and use of symptomology in determining exercise limits.

For asymptomatic, physically active young people modifications in intensity and duration of exercise are a simple matter involving minimal personal risks. Modifying an exercise prescription is more difficult for sedentary, older, or symptomatic participants. The degree of risk involved in exercise is a function of the interaction of: (1) the severity of the exercise relative to the habitual intensity of exercise performed, (2) age, (3) functional capacity, (4) health status, (5) risk factors for coronary heart disease and (6) symptomatology.

CARDIORESPIRATORY ENDURANCE ACTIVITIES

The intent of exercise prescription is to increase or maintain the functional capacity. To accomplish this goal a portion of each exercise session is devoted to aerobic endurance activities.

Endurance activities may be classified into two groups: Group 1 physical activities during which the exercise intensity is easily sustained with little variability in heart rate response (e.g. walking, jogging, running, swimming, cycling, cross-country skiing, and skating), and Group 2 physical activities during which continuous exercise intensity is not maintained (e.g. dancing, figure skating, mountain hiking, and a variety of games and sports).

When precise control of exercise intensity is necessary, as in the early stages of a conditioning or rehabilitation program, Group 1 activities are recommended. Individual fitness levels and personal preference determine whether Group 1 activities are performed in a continuous or discontinuous (interval conditioning) exercise format. These activities continue to be useful at all stages of a conditioning program because the participant is able to expend the most energy per unit time. Group 2 activities can be extremely useful because of the enjoyment provided in a physically active setting and the ability to direct the participant's attention away from anxieties, worries, and boredom.

Competitive aspects of games should be minimized to reduce the risk to participants. Modifications of game rules are often recommended. Such activities should not be included until participants obtain a minimal exercise intensity of 5 METs and the exercise leader becomes familiar with the physiologic and psychologic responses of the participants. Without modifications, competitive activities are not recommended for sedentary or multiple risk individuals. For asymptomatic sedentary participants a 6- to 10-week conditioning period will usually prepare a participant for most game activities. In addition to the exercise test, radio telemetry or ambulatory (Holter) ECG monitoring under actual exercise conditions may provide useful information about some diseased patients prior to their participation in self-regulated or recreational games.

INTENSITY OF EXERCISE

The most difficult problem in designing exercise programs is the prescription of the appropriate exercise intensity. This requires an individualized exercise prescription and adequate monitoring to ensure that the maximum prescribed intensity is not exceeded. The intensity of exercise may be expressed as a percentage of functional capacity. The percentage of functional capacity a given individual is able to sustain for a specified conditioning period is quite variable. Marathon runners are able to maintain 80% of functional capacity for over 2 hours, but poorly conditioned individuals exercising at 80% are fatigued in a few minutes. Such differences in the ability of persons to sustain a given exercise intensity must be taken into consideration in developing the exercise prescription.

Intensity of exercise during conditioning sessions should not be prescribed to exceed 85% of the functional capacity nor should it usually be lower than 50%. The average conditioning intensity for asymptomatic adults is usually between 60 and 70%. Participants, including cardiac patients, who have a low functional capacity, may initiate their conditioning at 40 to 60% of their functional capacity. Duration can then be set empirically, based on the individual responses, i.e., the participant should feel rested and not fatigued within an hour following exercise. The intensity of the exercise may be prescribed by heart rate, relative perceived exertion (RPE) or by METs.

Exercise Prescription by Heart Rate

In general, unless disturbed by environmental conditions, psychologic stimuli or disease, a linear relationship exists between heart rate and exercise intensity. Individual differences in the heart rate-exercise intensity relationship will be detected during the exercise test. The first method for calculating exercise heart rate is to plot the line that shows the relationship between the exercise heart rate and exercise intensity in either METs or $\dot{V}O_2$. The "maximal" heart rate is usually the heart rate measured at the highest exercise intensity attained. From this relationship, the heart rate associated with a given percentage of functional capacity (usually 60 to 70%) can be determined. This heart rate value, called the "target" heart rate, may be used for regulating intensity during conditioning.

A second method is to determine the target heart rate for a participant by multiplying the difference between the maximal and resting rates (heart rate range or reserve) by a percentage established on the basis of the functional capacity expressed in METs. This sliding scale accounts for the known effect of functional capacity on the relative exercise intensity that can be tolerated. The baseline intensity is set at 60% of the heart rate range and is adjusted upward in proportion to functional capacity. Thus, for persons with functional capacities ranging from 3 to 20 METs average conditioning intensity may be computed as follows:

Functional capacity (METs)	*Percentage of heart rate range*
3	60 + 3 = 63
5	60 + 5 = 65
*10	*60 + 10 = 70
15	60 + 15 = 75
20	60 + 20 = 80

The percentage of heart rate range computed above is then added to the resting heart rate to obtain the target heart rate. For example:

Maximal heart rate (beats per minute)		180
Resting heart rate		−60
		120
Conditioning intensity (% HR range)	* ×	.70
		84
Resting heart rate		+60
Average training heart rate		144

A third method for determining target heart rate is to calculate a specified percentage of the maximal HR. If the maximal HR is 180 beats per minute, the target heart rate might be 70% of 180 = (180 × .70) = 126 beats per minute. For a given percentage the first two methods for calculating target heart rate give similar results, but the third method underestimates the target heart rate for a given MET level by approximately 15%, and must be adjusted by adding 15% to the target heart rate calculated.

For practical purposes, the target heart rates calculated by the procedures outlined above are applicable to all the physical activities in which the individual may engage and under most environmental conditions. In discontinuous exercise the alternating higher and lower energy demands may be accompanied by heart rates 10% higher or 10% lower than the prescribed target heart rate. However, the exercise intervals should be of such duration that the heart rate, over time, averages out to the prescribed level.

Heart rate can be determined from measurements made during ECG monitoring, radiotelemetry, or palpation. The latter two methods are more adaptable to non-laboratory situations, with the palpation technique better suited to large groups. Counting the pulse for 10 (or 15) seconds immediately after a bout of exercise and multiplying by 6 (or 4) gives a good estimate of exercise heart rate.

Exercise Prescription by Rating of Perceived Exertion (RPE)

The RPE scale devised by Borg is shown in Chapter 2. It is a 15-point numerical scale ranging from 6 to 20 with a verbal description provided at every odd number. The RPE response to graded exercise correlates highly with cardiorespiratory and metabolic variables such as $\dot{V}O_2$, heart rate, ventilation and blood lactate concentration. RPE is a valid and reliable indicator of the level of physical exertion during constant intensity exercise and, therefore, can be used to establish an exercise intensity for endurance training.

Using the Borg scale, a perceived exertion rating of 12 to 13 corresponds to approximately 60% of the heart rate range. A rating of 15 corresponds to approximately 90% of heart rate range. Consequently most participants should exercise at an intensity rated between 12 and 15 (“somewhat hard” to “hard”).

The individual participant’s RPE response to graded exercise may be employed by specifying the RPE level for conditioning. Also, RPE can be used in conjunction with heart rate prescription methods. At the onset of a training program the participant can be instructed to exercise at a specified heart rate and to self-monitor the RPE at that intensity. Once the participant has developed a knowledge of the heart rate-RPE relationship, heart rate can be monitored less frequently and RPE can be employed as the primary method for regulating intensity. In addition, changes in RPE can be used as a guideline in modifying the exercise prescription.

Exercise Prescription by METs

The intensity of exercise may be prescribed by determining a specified percentage (50 to 85%) of the individual’s functional capacity and then selecting activities that are known to require energy expenditure at the desired level(s). Generally, 60 to 70% of functional capacity (maximal METs) is an appropriate average conditioning intensity.

The sliding scale procedure, as described with the heart rate method, can be employed when designating exercise intensity in terms of METs. The baseline intensity is set at 60% of the functional capacity in METs. Thus, for persons with functional capacities ranging from 3 to 20 METs:

Functional Capacity (METs)	*Computation of Percentage of Functional Capacity*	*Average Conditioning Intensity (METs)*
3	60 + 3 = 63	(.63 × 3 =) 1.90
5	60 + 5 = 65	3.25
10	60 + 10 = 70	7.00
15	60 + 15 = 75	11.25
20	60 + 20 = 80	16.00

Table 3–1 provides means and ranges for MET requirements of many of the common leisure activities. Appendix D also contains information on energy costs of selected activities.

Regardless of the prescriptive technique employed, the average exercise intensity during a given conditioning session may be obtained by alternating periods of exercise at higher and lower intensities. If, for example, an exercise intensity of 5.5 METs (or comparable heart rate or RPE) is prescribed, equal time intervals at 4 and 7 METs will result in the prescribed 5.5 MET average. Thus, any modification can be prescribed precisely. Usually the initial exercise prescription should set exercise intensity about 1 MET lower than the target until the participant has become accustomed to exercise and the exercise leader is familiar with the participant's response. Generally, peak conditioning intensity should not exceed 85% of functional capacity.

For physical activities such as walking, jogging, running, cycle ergometer exercise, and stepping or stair climbing, the exercise intensity in METs is directly related to speed of movement, measurable resistance, or mass lifted (see Appendix D). Even in these activities, the maintenance of the prescribed safe conditioning intensity can be complicated by changes in the environment. Critical environmental factors include: wind, hills, sand, snow, obstacles such as ditches, fences or underbrush, heat or cold, humidity, altitude, pollution, bulky clothing or clothing that obstructs movement, and the weight and size of equipment such as back packs, skis, suitcases, or grocery bags. The problem of exercising at a prescribed conditioning intensity in any activity under most environmental conditions may be solved by using heart rate as an indicator of exercise

Table 3–1. Leisure Activities in METS: Sports, Exercise Classes, Games, Dancing

	Mean	*Range*
Archery	3.9	3–4
Back Packing	—	5–11
Badminton	5.8	4–9+
Basketball		
Gameplay	8.3	7–12+
Non-game	—	3–9
Billiards	2.5	–
Bowling	—	2–4
Boxing		
In-ring	13.3	–
Sparring	8.3	–
Canoeing, Rowing and Kayaking	—	3–8
Conditioning Exercise	—	3–8+
Climbing Hills	7.2	5–10+
Cricket	5.2	4.6–7.4
Croquet	3.5	–
Cycling		
Pleasure or to work	—	3–8+
10 mph	7.0	–
Dancing (Social, Square, Tap)	—	3.7–7.4
Dancing (Aerobic)	—	6–9
Fencing	—	6–10+
Field Hockey	8.0	–
Fishing		
from bank	3.7	2–4
wading in stream	—	5–6
Football (Touch)	7.9	6–10
Golf		
Power cart	—	2–3
Walking (carrying bag or pulling cart)	5.1	4–7
Handball	—	8–12+
Hiking (Cross-country)	—	3–7
Horseback Riding		
Galloping	8.2	–
Trotting	6.6	–
Walking	2.4	–

Table 3–1. Leisure Activities in METS: Sports, Exercise Classes, Games, Dancing *Continued*

	Mean	*Range*
Horseshoe Pitching	—	2–3
Hunting (Bow or Gun)		
Small game (walking, carrying light load)	—	3–7
Big game (dragging carcass, walking)	—	3–14
Judo	13.5	–
Mounting Climbing	—	5–10+
Music Playing	—	2–3
Paddleball, Racquetball	9	8–12
Rope Jumping	11	–
60–80 skips/min	9	–
120–140 skips/min	—	11–12
Running		
12 min per mile	8.7	–
11 min per mile	9.4	–
10 min per mile	10.2	–
9 min per mile	11.2	–
8 min per mile	12.5	–
7 min per mile	14.1	–
6 min per mile	16.3	–
Sailing	—	2–5
Scubadiving	—	5–10
Shuffleboard	—	2–3
Skating, Ice and Roller	—	5–8
Skiing, Snow		
Downhill	—	5–8
Crosscountry	—	6–12+
Skiing, Water	—	5–7
Sledding, Tobogganing	—	4–8
Snowshoeing	9.9	7–14
Squash	—	8–12+
Soccer	—	5–12+
Stairclimbing	—	4–8
Swimming	—	4–8+
Table Tennis	4.1	3–5
Tennis	6.5	4–9+
Volleyball	—	3–6

intensity. Prescription and maintenance of safe exercise intensities are more difficult in complex dual sports such as tennis, handball, or squash, and team sports such as volleyball, softball, soccer, or basketball.

In a specific physical conditioning session, the exercise leader may use the MET prescription, heart rate prescription, RPE prescription or all in setting appropriate exercise intensities in various activities. As one adapts to conditioning, heart rate and RPE for a given MET level generally decrease; therefore, participants should increase their MET level progressively to correspond to their target heart rate or RPE. Periodic re-evaluation aids in measuring progress and updating the exercise prescription.

With regard to prescription of exercise intensity it is important to remember that intensity should be prescribed within a range regardless of the method used. For example, if the percentage of heart rate range method is used, and a target heart rate of 144 is calculated, one should expect a participant's exercise heart rate to vary around that number. For various reasons some individuals will not be able to comfortably tolerate the work load, others might find it much too easy. It is reasonable to expect the exercise to vary by about 10% of the calculated target. Adjusting the individual's exercise heart rate within this range is part of the art of exercise leadership.

Finally, it should be emphasized that the individual's signs and symptoms of CHD or other disease may be overriding factors in prescribing the intensity of exercise. As will be discussed in Chapters 4 and 5, certain manifestations of chronic disease (e.g., angina pectoris, intermittant claudication, chronic obstructive pulmonary disease) may require that exercise intensity be maintained at levels below those calculated using the standard procedures described above.

DURATION OF THE EXERCISE SESSION

The conditioning period, exclusive of warm-up and cool down, may vary in length from 15 to 60 minutes. Most typically the conditioning phase is 20 to 30 minutes. This length of time is required to improve functional capacity. The appropriate duration of the conditioning period is inversely related to the intensity of the exercise expressed as a percentage of the functional capacity. Compared to persons with low functional capacities, individuals with high functional capacities are able to maintain higher intensity exercise for a longer period of time. The conditioning response resulting from an exercise program is a result of the product of the intensity and the duration of exercise (total energy expenditure). Significant cardiovascular improvements have been obtained with exercise sessions of 5 to 10 minutes' duration with an intensity of more than 90% of functional capacity. However, high intensity-short duration sessions are not desirable for most sedentary or symptomatic participants and better results are obtained with lower intensities and longer durations. Such programs are preferred because they carry lower risk of orthopedic injury and involve a relatively high total caloric expenditure.

For sedentary, asymptomatic, and symptomatic participants exercise sessions of moderate duration (20 to 30 minutes) and moderate intensity (40 to 70% of functional capacity) are advisable during the first weeks of conditioning. Changes in the exercise prescription may be made as the individual's functional capacity increases and as physiologic adaptation to exercise occurs. Modification of the duration-intensity level should be individualized on the basis of the subject's functional capacity, health status, and response to specific exercise activities. If a normal conditioning response is obtained with no complications, the duration may be increased gradually from 20 to 45 minutes after the first 2 weeks. As mentioned previously, the interaction of intensity and duration should be such that the participant has no undue fatigue an hour after the completion of the exercise session.

FREQUENCY OF EXERCISE SESSIONS

The frequency of exercise depends in part on the duration and intensity of the exercise session. The frequency varies from several daily sessions, to 3 to 7 periods per week according to the needs, interests and functional capacity of the participants. For some individuals with functional capacities less than 3 METs, sessions of 5 minutes several times daily may be desirable. For persons with capacities between 3 and 5 METs, 1 to 2 daily sessions may be advisable. Participants with capacities of 5 to 8 METs should exercise at least 3 times per week on alternate days.

When initiating a jogging program, excessive bone-joint stress may occur. It is desirable to alternate a day of exercise with a day of rest. Once adaptation is accomplished a greater conditioning response may be obtained with daily exercise.

RATE OF PROGRESSION

Progression in the exercise conditioning program is dependent on an individual's functional capacity, health status, age, and needs or goals. The endurance or aerobic phase of the exercise prescription has three stages of progression: initial, improvement, and maintenance.

Initial Conditioning Stage

The initial stage should include stretching, light calisthenics, and low level aerobic activities with which the participant experiences a minimum of muscle soreness and avoids debilitating injuries or discomfort. Discomfort is often associated with starting an exercise program without adequate time for physiologic adaptation. Program adherence may be reduced if a program is initiated too abruptly. It may help to start with an exercise intensity approximately 1 MET lower than that estimated at 50 to 85% of the functional capacity. By using the graded exercise test results and the calculated exercise intensity in METs, the exercise specialist, health fitness instructor, health fitness director, or exercise program director can estimate the aerobic phase exercise intensity for different types of activities. For example, an exercise intensity of an eventual 7 to 9 METs at a target rate of 144 to 168, might be set initially at a more conservative 6 METs. If the participant selects a jogging program, information in Appendix D indicates that a 4 mph pace would be appropriate. A cycle ergometer program might also be suggested for this 70 kg participant at 600 kg m min^{-1}. These estimates of intensity should always be checked by having the participant, unless symptom limited, exercise at these intensities for a minimum of 3 minutes and then checking the pulse. Exercise intensities may require adjustment; lower intensity if the participant is above the target heart rate, and higher intensity if the participant is below the target heart rate. With conditioning, heart rate decreases for a given exercise intensity. Therefore, the heart rate (used in combination with signs and symptoms) is one of the best indicators of when to advance the participant to the next level. A combination of objective and subjective factors must be considered when progressing individuals in their exercise routines.

The total duration of the initial exercise phase of the exercise prescription should be at least 10 to 15 minutes and should be gradually increased. Frequency depends on the initial functional capacity (Table 3–2). The initial phase usually lasts from 4 to 6 weeks, but this is dependent on the adaptation of the participant to the program. For example, a person who has a fitness level ranked "fair" or who is limited by CHD may spend as many as 6 to 10 weeks in the initial program, while the participant with a fitness level of "good to high" may not need to participate as long in the initial phase or may be exempted from this stage if already engaged in an exercise program.

Health status must also be considered in the rate of progression. For example, patients with symptoms of exertional angina during the initial stage may have to exercise for a period of time at 40 to 50% of functional capacity. Persons with intermittent claudication may only be able to tolerate 1 to 2 minutes of exercise alternated with rest periods. Following a debilitating illness or major surgical procedure functional capacities are often as low as 2 to 3 METs. Initially, exercise duration may be less than 5 minutes due to angina, local muscle fatigue, or breathlessness. The necessity for individual modifications cannot be overemphasized, although no attempt can be made to provide a list of all the possible modifications for all participants. More detail on this issue is provided in Chapters 4 and 5.

Improvement Conditioning Stage

The improvement stage of the aerobic phase of the exercise conditioning program differs from the initial stage in that the participant is progressed at a more rapid rate. During this stage intensity is increased to the targeted level within the 50 to 85 range of functional capacity. Duration is increased consistently every 2 to 3 weeks. How well the participant adapts to the

Table 3–2. Cardiorespiratory Fitness Levels*

Fitness Level	*O_2 ml/kg · min*	*METS*
Poor	3.5–13.9	1.0– 3.9
Low	14.0–24.9	4.0– 6.9
Average	25.0–38.9	7.0–10.9
Good	39.0–48.9	11.0–13.9
High	49.0–56.0	14.0–16.0

*For 40-year-old males. Adjustments are appropriate to apply these standards to others.

current level of conditioning dictates the frequency and magnitude of the increments. Cardiac patients and less fit individuals should be permitted more time for adaptation at each stage of conditioning. It is recommended that symptom limited participants initially use discontinuous aerobic exercise and progress toward continuous aerobic exercise. The duration of exercise for these participants should be increased to 20 to 30 minutes before increasing the intensity (Table 3–3).

Age must also be taken into consideration when progressions are recommended. Experience suggests that adaptation to conditioning may take longer in older individuals.

Maintenance Conditioning Stage

The maintenance stage of the exercise prescription usually begins after the first 6 months of training. During the maintenance stage the participant usually reaches a satisfactory level of cardiorespiratory fitness and may be no longer interested in increasing the conditioning load. While further improvement may be minimal, continuing the same workout schedule enables one to maintain fitness.

At this point, the objectives of conditioning should be reviewed and realistic goals set. To maintain fitness, a specific exercise program should be designed that will be similiar in energy cost to the conditioning program and also satisfy the needs of the participant over a long time span. More enjoyable or variable activities may be substituted for the improvement stage activities of walking and jogging. This may help avoid participant dropout which often results when activities become boring due to repetition.

BODY COMPOSITION

Obesity, an excessive percentage of body fat (% fat), is associated with increased risk for development of hypertension, diabetes, coronary heart disease and other chronic diseases. In addition, obesity often carries a negative social stigma and is associated with a reduced physical working capacity. Many participants in preventive and rehabilitative exercise programs are excessively fat. Since normalization of body composition is a need and/or a goal of many exercise program participants, exercise prescriptions should be designed to aid in accomplishing this end. This section presents the principles that should be employed in modifying body composition.

Table 3–3. Example: Progression of the Symptomatic Participant Using a Discontinuous Aerobic Conditioning Phase*

Endurance/ Aerobic Phase	*Weeks*	*Total Minutes at % FC***	*% FC*	*Minutes at Exercise Intensity (60–80% FC)*	*Minutes at Rest Phase Lower than Exercise Intensity*	*Repetitions*
	1	12	60	2	1	6
	2	14	60	2	1	7
Initial Stage	3	16	60	2	1	8
	4	18	60–70	2	1	9
	5	20	60–70	2	1	10
	6–9	21	70–80	3	1	7
	10–13	24	70–80	3	1	8
Improvement Stage	14–16	24	70–80	4	1	6
	17–19	28	70–80	4	1	7
	20–23	30	70–80	5	1	6
	24–27	30	70–80	Continuous		
Maintenance Stage	28+	45–60	70–80	Continuous		

*Clinical status must be considered before advancing to the next level
**FC—Functional Capacity

CALORIC BALANCE

Body composition is determined by a complex set of genetic and behavioral factors. Though the contributing variables are many, the fundamental determinant of body weight and body composition is caloric balance. Caloric balance refers to the ratio between caloric intake (energy equivalent of food ingested) and caloric expenditure (energy equivalent of biological work performed). Body weight is lost when caloric expenditure exceeds caloric intake (negative balance) and weight is gained when the opposite situation exists. Though it is predictable that shifts in caloric balance will be accompanied by changes in body weight, the nature of a weight change varies markedly with the specific behaviors that lead to a caloric imbalance. For example, fasting and extreme caloric restriction diets cause substantial losses of water and lean tissue. In contrast, an exercise-induced negative caloric balance results in weight losses that consist primarily of adipose tissue. High resistance programs (e.g. weight lifting) may lead to a gain in lean weight, while aerobic training usually results only in a maintenance of lean weight. Both types of programs can contribute to a loss of fat.

PROPER WEIGHT LOSS PROGRAMS

Substantial evidence indicates that, for most persons, the optimal approach to weight loss combines a mild caloric restriction with regular endurance exercise. The American College of Sports Medicine (*Med Science Sports Exercise 15*: IX–XIII, 1983) has stated that a desirable weight loss program is one that:

1. Provides intake not lower than 1200 $kcal \cdot d^{-1}$ for normal adults in order to get a proper blend of foods to meet nutritional requirements. (Note: this requirement may change for children, older individuals, athletes, etc).
2. Includes foods acceptable to the dieter in terms of sociocultural background, usual habits, taste, costs and ease in acquisition and preparation.
3. Provides a negative caloric balance (not to exceed 500–1000 $kcal \cdot d^{-1}$ lower than recommended) resulting in gradual weight loss without metabolic derangements. Maximal weight loss should be 1 $kg \cdot wk^{-1}$.
4. Includes the use of behavior modification techniques to

identify and eliminate diet habits that contribute to improper nutrition.

5. Includes an endurance exercise program of at least 3 $d \cdot wk^{-1}$, 20 to 30 minutes in duration, at a minimum intensity of 65% of maximal heart rate.
6. Provides that the new eating and physical activity habits can be continued for life in order to maintain the achieved lower body weight.

Weight loss programs that manifest the aforementioned characteristics have been shown to minimize the nutritional deficiencies and losses of fat-free tissue that result from severe restrictions of caloric intake.

In designating the exercise component of a weight loss regimen, the principles presented earlier in this chapter should be employed. Sustained aerobic activities cause the greatest total caloric expenditure; however CHD or other disease may be overriding factors in prescribing primarily by the total work output. Therefore, when exercise is prescribed for the primary purpose of promoting weight loss, the ratio between intensity and duration of exercise should be regulated so as to yield a high total caloric expenditure (200 to 500 kcal per session for adults). Obese individuals are at an increased relative risk for orthopedic injury. This may require that the intensity of exercise be maintained at or below the 65% of maximal heart rate recommended for improvement of cardiorespiratory endurance. Non-weight bearing activities may be necessary. Adaptation in frequency and duration may also be required.

A minimal energy expenditure of 300 kcal per exercise session and 1000 kcal per week is recommended for both asymptomatic and symptomatic participants. The average healthy sedentary participant (8 to 12 METs functional capacity) can usually attain the 200 kcal level per exercise session during the first week of conditioning. The average participant with a steady progression can reach 300 kcal per exercise session in 8 to 12 weeks, while some cardiac patients or other symptomatic participants may require as long as 2 years. The difference between the two groups is due to the greater variability in myocardial limitations rather than in their adaptation to conditioning. Usually, increased frequency of conditioning of up to 5 to 6 days per week is desirable and greatly increases the total energy expenditure.

FLEXIBILITY

Normal musculoskeletal function requires that an adequate range of motion be maintained in all joints. Of particular concern is maintenance of flexibility in the lower back/posterior thigh region. Lack of flexibility in this region is associated with the increased risk for development of chronic lower back pain. Therefore, preventive and rehabilitative exercise programs should include activities that promote maintenance of good flexibility, particularly in the lower back.

Stretching exercise can aid in improving and maintaining range of motion in a joint or series of joints. Flexibility exercises should be performed slowly with a gradual progression to greater ranges of motion. A slow dynamic movement should be followed with a static stretch that is sustained for 10 to 30 seconds. The degree of stretch should not be so extreme as to cause significant pain. Stretching exercises should be performed at least 3 times per week and can be effectively included in the warm-up and/or cool-down periods that precede and follow the aerobic conditioning phase of an exercise session.

The musculoskeletal injuries associated with jogging and running often can be avoided by performing stretching exercises for the posterior thigh and lower leg muscles. Moderate static stretching exercise also may be useful to relieve neuromuscular tension.

MUSCULAR STRENGTH AND ENDURANCE

Muscular strength and endurance have little direct relationship to cardiorespiratory fitness or functional capacity. However, many leisure and occupational tasks require arm exercises, e.g. moving, lifting or holding a weight. The physiologic stress induced by lifting or holding a given weight is proportional to the percentage of maximal strength involved. The maintenance or enhancement of muscle strength and muscle endurance enables the individual to perform such tasks with less physiologic stress. Maintenance of adequate strength becomes an increasingly important issue with advancing age which is associated with a loss of lean weight.

Muscular strength is acquired either by dynamic high-tension low-repetition exercises or through static contractions. Both dynamic lifting procedures and static contractions result in an increased systemic arterial blood pressure. An increased blood pressure increases the work of the heart and its requirements for oxygen. Such lifts may cause a reduction in venous return and result in decreased blood flow to the heart and brain if performed with the Valsalva maneuver. Maximal tension exercises should be discouraged for symtomatic or high risk individuals. Instead, dynamic low-weight exercises should be incorporated into the program for improvement of both muscle strength and endurance. If such activities are used, participants should be trained to make all strength movements while breathing freely without breath-holding. Exhalation on effort should be encouraged. In addition, special attention must be directed toward sufficient warm-up and cool-down, correct structural and functional body position for lifting, and rhythmic performance of the necessary movements.

Strengthening exercises should be performed 3 times per week. Resistance may be applied to the muscles using free-weights, supported weight machines or calisthenic exercises. Optimal rates of strength gain can occur when resistance is established at a level that allows no more than 5 to 7 repetitions of a movement and when three sets of the exercise are performed in a training session. However, significant strength gains can occur with exercises that apply lower levels of resistance (e.g. calisthenic exercises). It should be emphasized that high resistances are to be avoided with high risk, symptomatic and CHD patients.

ENVIRONMENTAL FACTORS

The physiologic responses to exercise may be profoundly affected by environmental factors such as extreme heat or cold, high altitude and air pollution. As the exercise environment varies, the exercise prescription should be modified so that physiologic responses remain at the desired levels and the participant's health and safety are maintained. The exercise heart rate is a useful method of adjusting intensity for varying environmental conditions.

Environmental heat stress is a function of temperature, relative humidity and radiant heating. Increased heat stress characteristically involves a greater sweat rate and cardiorespiratory response to a standard submaximal exercise load. Therefore, maintenance of a constant cardiorespiratory response necessitates a decrease in absolute work intensity. In extremely warm conditions duration of exercise should be restricted and care should be taken to adequately replace fluids during and after the exercise session. In extremely cold conditions the exerciser should provide protection against frost bite. Clothing should be worn that adequately protects the head and extremities. Whenever possible, symptomatic and high risk exercisers should exercise in moderate temperatures.

At high altitudes the partial pressure of oxygen in atmospheric air is reduced. This can impair systemic oxygen transport and cause an increased cardiorespiratory response to a standard submaximal exercise intensity. Therefore, upon ascent to higher altitudes (1500 meters +) the exercise prescription should be modified by decreasing the absolute exercise intensity.

High levels of air pollution may necessitate a restriction of the intensity and/or duration of exercise. This is of particular importance for patients with chronic pulmonary disease.

THE EXERCISE SESSION

Each exercise session includes a warm-up, 5 to 10 minutes; endurance (aerobic) activity, 15 to 60 minutes; cool-down, 5 to 10 minutes. The warm-up period is designed to gradually increase the metabolic rate from the resting level of 1 MET to the MET level required for conditioning. The warm-up period usually lasts 5 to 10 minutes and includes stretching exercises (joint-readiness), calisthenics or other types of muscle conditioning exercises, walking or slow jogging. The duration and intensity of each of these activities depends on environmental conditions, functional capacity, symptomatology, and exercise preference of the participant. For participants who require or prefer greater amounts of muscle strength or endurance, additional calisthenics and exercises utilizing weights may be included (10 to 20 minutes). However, moderate to heavy lifting activities or exercising with weights are not recommended for persons with hypertension, arrhythmias, or poor cardiac reserve. The endurance or aerobic phase of conditioning can be designed to be continuous or discontinuous. It includes aerobic-type activities involving large muscle groups to produce heart rates of prescribed intensity. The cool-down period includes exercises of diminishing intensities, e.g. slower walking or jogging, stretching and in some cases, relaxation activities. Also, the exercise session may appropriately include a period of participation in recreational games.

PROGRAM SUPERVISION

Medical evaluation and exercise testing permit the classification of participants according to their capacity for participation in an unsupervised or supervised exercise program.

UNSUPERVISED EXERCISE PROGRAMS

Apparently healthy participants with functional capacities of 8 METS or more can usually exercise safely in an unsupervised conditioning program. Participant safety can be enhanced by provision of an individualized exercise prescription and participant awareness of the physiologic effects of temperature, humidity, and altitude.

SUPERVISED EXERCISE PROGRAMS

A supervised exercise program is one that provides trained professional on-site leadership (e.g. health fitness instructor or exercise specialist). Such a program is recommended for high risk, symptomatic and cardiorespiratory patients who are considered by their physicians to be clinically stable and who have been cleared by their physician for participation in the program. Also, supervised programs are initially advisable for asymptomatic participants with functional capacities less than 8 METs. Although a signed informed consent may not be required, it may be useful in communicating the attendent risks and benefits of exercise.

MEDICALLY SUPERVISED EXERCISE PROGRAMS

A medically supervised exercise program provides direct physician supervision or is supervised by trained professional leaders who are authorized to deliver defibrillation and to administer daily exercises. Such programs are recommended for; (1) cardiorespiratory patients who are initiating an exercise program, (2) patients who manifest unstable clinical profiles, and (3) high risk, symptomatic or chronic disease patients whose personal physician feels that medical supervision is required to ensure participant safety. Informed consent must be obtained in medically supervised programs (Appendix C).

REFERENCES

American College of Sports Medicine. Position statement on the recommended quantity and quality of exercise for developing and maintaining fitness in healthy adults. *Med Sci Sports 10*:vii–x, 1978.

American College of Sports Medicine. Position statement on proper and improper weight loss programs. *Med Sci Sports Exer 15*:ix–xiii, 1983.

Committee on Exercise. *Exercise Testing and Training of Apparently Healthy Individuals: A Handbook for Physicians.* New York: American Heart Association, 1972.

Melleby, A: *The Y's Way to a Healthy Back.* Piscataway, NJ: New Century Publishers, 1982.

Noble BJ: Clinical applications of perceived exertion. *Med Sci Sports Exer 14*:406–411, 1982.

Pollock ML: How much exercise is enough? *Phys Sportsmed. 6*:50–64, 1978.

Pollock ML, Wilmore JH and Fox SM: *Exercise in Health and Disease.* Philadelphia: WB Saunders Co., 1984.

4

Exercise Prescription for Cardiac Patients

Cardiac rehabilitation is a multiphasic program of medical care that is designed to restore the coronary heart diseased (CHD) patient to a full and productive life. Programs are concerned with the physiologic, psychologic, social, vocational and recreational aspects of human function. The following intervention modules are included in many cardiac rehabilitation programs: exercise therapy, psychologic counseling, vocational counseling, and patient education/behavior modification regimens to facilitate dietary change, smoking cessation and stress management. All programs provide medical surveillance of the rehabilitating patient. In recent years, exercise training has become a widely accepted therapeutic modality for CHD patients and has become a central focus in many cardiac rehabilitation programs. The general principles of exercise prescription as discussed in Chapter 3 apply to CHD patients as well as to healthy persons. However, the physiologic limitations imposed by CHD require that particular care be taken to individualize the exercise prescription in accordance with the patient's health history and clinical status. This chapter is designed to present the guidelines that should be employed in prescribing exercise for cardiac patients of various classes. The material in this chapter has been organized by dividing the rehabilitative process into *three* major phases: Inpatient (Phase I), Outpatient (Phase II), and Community programs (Phase III). However, it is recognized that cardiac rehabilitation programs can appropriately be divided into four or more phases.

TYPES OF CARDIAC PATIENTS

Cardiac patients vary in severity of atherosclerotic disease, impairment of ventricular function, functional capacity, occurrence of signs and symptoms, and clinical manifestations of disease (e.g., ischemia, abnormal blood pressure response). A rehabilitation program may include patients who have had coronary artery bypass surgery, myocardial infarction, pacemaker implantation, valve replacement, or coronary angioplasty; or who have other evidence of cardiovascular disease such as angina pectoris or a positive exercise test, or other evidence of disease from a radionuclide study or coronary cathertization. Emphasis should be placed on developing goals for recovery of the patients that are realistic and consistent with limitations imposed by the disease process. When designing the exercise prescription consideration should be given to the patient's stage of convalescence and individual needs. Caution and discretion should be used in prescribing the intensity of exercise. Considerations should be given to signs and symptoms that may occur with increased duration of exercise at a set intensity and with limitations due to changes in medications or orthopedic/neuromuscular problems that may become apparent with exercise training. An initial exercise prescription should be confirmed only after closely monitoring the patient's responses to the prescription. Adjustments may be required to align target heart rate and predicted exercise intensity (i.e., METs, pace).

INPATIENT EXERCISE PROGRAMS (PHASE I)

The inpatient exercise program is frequently offered for post-myocardial infarction, postoperative cardiovascular, pulmonary disease, peripheral vascular disease patients and other patient groups that may benefit from such services while in the hospital. The inpatient program usually includes supervised ambulatory therapy. The staff-patient ratio is generally 1:1. ECG monitoring equipment must be available for determining appropriate exercise responses and an emergency team should be available on the premise. The goals of the inpatient exercise program are to provide medical surveillance of patients, to return patients to daily physical activities, to offset the deleterious physiologic and psychologic effects of bedrest and to prepare patients for stages of cardiac rehabilitation that will follow. The goals of the program should be individualized to the needs of the patient. Those patients who have been quite sedentary (e.g., some elderly patients) may require only an exercise program that allows them to return to activities of daily living (ADL). Other patients may be strong candidates for tertiary prevention activities and may begin lifelong programs to improve cardiorespiratory endurance, body composition, flexibility and muscular strength/endurance.

EXERCISE PRESCRIPTION METHODS

Contraindications for inpatients participating in ambulatory exercise are given in Table 4–1. Presence or development of these special problems may require temporary delay of initiation or discontinuance of the exercise program until the appropriate medical management has alleviated the problem.

Termination points for an inpatient exercise session are generally more conservative than those outlined for terminating an outpatient session or exercise test (Table 4–2). Further diagnostic evaluation of the patient is warranted if any of the following signs or symptoms occur during the inpatient exercise session: increased heart rate above the prescribed limit, myocardial ischemia, significant arrhythmias, angina pectoris, incisional pain, or excessive fatigue.

In the initial phase (1 to 3 days post myocardial infarction or surgical procedure) of the inpatient program, activities should be restricted to low intensity (approximately 2 to 3 METs). Generally, these consist of self-care activities and se-

Table 4–1. Contraindications for Entry into Inpatient and Outpatient Exercise Programs

The following criteria may be used as contraindications for program entry.

1. Unstable angina.
2. Resting systolic blood pressure over 200 mm Hg or resting diastolic blood pressure over 100 mm Hg.
3. Significant drop (20 mm Hg or more) in resting systolic blood pressure from the patient's average level which cannot be explained by medications.
4. Moderate to severe aortic stenosis.
5. Acute systemic illness or fever.
6. Uncontrolled atrial or ventricular arrhythmias.
7. Uncontrolled tachycardia (greater than 100 bpm).
8. Symptomatic congestive heart failure.
9. Third degree heart block.
10. Active pericarditis or myocarditis.
11. Recent embolism.
12. Thrombophlebitis.
13. Resting ST displacement (greater than 3 mm)
14. Uncontrolled diabetes.
15. Orthopedic problems that would prohibit exercise.

Table 4–2. Criteria for Termination of an Inpatient Exercise Session

The following guidelines may be used to terminate the exercise session for cardiac inpatients:

1. Fatigue.
2. Failure of monitoring equipment.
3. Light-headedness, confusion, ataxia, pallor, cyanosis, dyspnea, nausea, or any peripheral circulatory insufficiency.
4. Onset of angina with exercise.
5. Symptomatic supraventricular tachycardia.
6. ST displacement (greater than 3 mm horizontal or down sloping from rest).
7. Ventricular tachycardia (3 or more consecutive PVCs).
8. Exercise induced left or right bundle branch block.
9. Onset of second and/or third degree heart block.
10. R on T PVCs (one).
11. Frequent unifocal PVCs (greater than 30% of the complexes).
12. Frequent multifocal PVCs (greater than 30% of the complexes).
13. Couplets (greater than 2 per minute).
14. Increase in heart rate over 20 bpm above standing resting heart rate for MI patients.
15. Drop of 10 mm Hg or more in systolic blood pressure.
16. Excessive blood pressure rise: systolic greater than or equal to 220 or diastolic greater than or equal to 110 mm Hg.
17. Inappropriate bradycardia (drop in heart rate greater than 10 bpm) with increase or no change in work load.

lected arm and leg exercises designed to maintain muscle tone, reduce orthostatic hypotension, and maintain joint mobility. These exercises should be progressed from lying to sitting and then standing. Eventually (3 to 5 days post event) walking, treadmill or stationary cycle ergometery may be added. Although the inpatient exercise session may follow the pattern of warm-up, endurance aerobic activity, and cool-down, exercise sessions may be as short as 5 to 10 minutes per session. As specified in Chapter 3, exercise intensity may be set as low as 40 to 60% of the patient's functional capacity. However, functional capacity of the inpatient may not be known and, in such cases, should be assumed to be quite low (3 to 5 METs).

Although heart rate may be a useful technique for prescribing exercise intensity with some in-patients, it may be impractical with others (e.g. patients with beta blocking and calcium channel blocking medications). Generally, standing resting heart rate plus 20 to 30 bpm or a perceived exertion of 12 to 13 on the Borg scale is an appropriate intensity index for use with in-patients. For those with a functional capacity estimated or measured at 3 to 5 METs, duration might be set at 5 to 10 minutes with 2 to 4 sessions performed per day. Those with lower functional capacities may require shorter duration and more frequent sessions per day (see Chapter 3). As duration is extended, frequency of exercise can be reduced. Duration of exercise should be gradually increased to 20 to 30 minutes 1 to 2 times daily and an exercise test should be conducted prior to increasing the exercise intensity to greater than 5 METs.

EXERCISE TESTING AND DISCHARGE PLANNING

Low-level pre-hospital discharge exercise testing of patients with acute myocardial infarction yields quantitative information regarding the ECG, hemodynamic changes or symptomatic responses to submaximal exercise. Such data provide information regarding patient status, which is particularly useful in formulating discharge planning and guidelines for resumption of ADL during early convalescence.

The intensity of the initial stages of predischarge exercise tests are generally lower than those for conventional protocols, although similar recording methods, monitoring procedures, supervision and safety precautions are used. The purpose of the low-level hospital exercise test is to determine the response of the patient to metabolic loads that are comparable to those that will be performed during early convalescence (i.e., self-care, walking, stair climbing), generally less than 5 METs. The criteria for terminating these tests are more rigorous than those for stopping maximal exercise tests. However, in the absence of specific signs and symptoms a patient may be tested to higher metabolic loads (> 5 METs) or to the symptom limited level.

Low-level exercise testing also provides indications for additional diagnostic studies (angiogram, isotopic evaluation) and therapeutic needs. For example, administration of antiarrhythmic or antianginal medications may be indicated for patients who demonstrate arrhythmias or significant ST segment depression during low-level testing.

Finally, certain responses to low-level exercise testing have been associated with poor patient prognosis. These include reduced functional capacity (less than 5 METs, a sensitive indicator of left ventricular function), malignant ventricular arrhythmias, significant ST segment depression or elevation, a low maximal systolic blood pressure (below 140 mm Hg), or an exercise induced decrease in systolic blood pressure.

In summary, low level exercise testing prior to hospital discharge provides valuable information to facilitate optimal clinical management and individualized prescriptions for medications and physical activities.

OUTPATIENT OR HOME EXERCISE PROGRAMS (PHASE II)

The Phase II cardiac rehabilitation exercise program provides a continuation of the inpatient program and usually begins immediately after hospital discharge. Ideally, the Phase II program should be administered on an outpatient basis in a hospital or other facility in which ECG monitoring, emergency support and direct professional supervision are available. In such programs staff-patient ratio may vary from 1:1 to 1:5 depending on the functional capacity, symptoms and ECG characteristics of patients involved. If an outpatient program is not available or feasible, the Phase II exercise program may be implemented by the patient at home or at a community-based facility. With home programs it is preferred that the patient periodically attend an outpatient program for monitored reevaluation. Regardless of site, the goal of the Phase II exercise program is to provide physical rehabilitation for resumption of habitual and occupational activities and to promote positive lifestyle changes. The program is operated under the direction of a physician who may be in attendance regularly with outpatient programs or who may be on call for home, community based or outpatient sessions.

EXERCISE PRESCRIPTION METHODS

The techniques used in prescribing exercise in Phase II programs vary with the functional capacity of the patient. In general, for patients with functional capacities of 5 METs or less the techniques discussed for inpatients are appropriate. For patients with functional capacities above 5 METs the prescriptive techniques using heart rate and ratings of perceived exertion as discussed in Chapter 3 are applicable. Frequency of exercise should be 3 to 4 sessions per week. Duration of exercise should be gradually increased from as little as 10 to 15 minutes to as much as 30 to 60 minutes as the functional capacity and clinical status improve.

CRITERIA FOR DISCHARGE FROM AN OUTPATIENT (PHASE II) PROGRAM

The duration of an outpatient program varies in accordance with local program guidelines but most programs start within 1 week of hospital discharge and last between 8 and 16 weeks prior to entrance into a maintenance or community (Phase III) program. Standard criteria for discharge from an outpatient program are not currently defined. However, the following criteria should be considered:

- *Functional capacity.* Since the patient's essential daily activities after hospital discharge require up to 3 METs, the patient should have a 5 MET capacity which will allow a safe range of metabolic reserve during sustained activity of up to 3 METs.
- *Medical status.* The medical status of the patient should be stable. The following criteria should be met:
  - — normal hemodynamic responses to exercise including appropriate increases in blood pressure, a normal or unchanged ECG at peak exercise with normal or unchanged conduction, arrhythmias stable or absent and a stable or medically acceptable ischemic response,
  - — angina stable or absent, and
  - — stable and/or controlled resting heart rate and blood pressure (i.e., less than 90 beats/min and 140/90, respectively).
- *Physical fitness.* The patient should have an adequate level of physical fitness (i.e., muscular strength, endurance, functional capacity and body composition) for daily activities and/or occupation.
- *Education.* Patients should have satisfactory understanding of the following:
  - — basic pathophysiology of their cardiovascular disease,
  - — rationale for the intervention approach being employed,
  - — lifestyle characteristics associated with low risk or coronary heart disease
  - — reason(s) for any prescribed cardiovascular medications and expected side-effects, and
  - — range of safe activities permitted including sexual activity and vocational and recreational pursuits.

In addition, patients should demonstrate an ability to maintain the exercise prescription within the designated range and to recognize signs and symptoms of exertional intolerance.

OUTPATIENT GROUP PROGRAMS VERSUS HOME PROGRAMS

Although it has been demonstrated that acute cardiac patients with nonischemic responses to treadmill exercise testing can safely undergo unsupervised exercise training at home, most authorities generally recommend that cardiac patients, at least initially, exercise in a group setting under medical supervision.

Group outpatient exercise programs, particularly during early convalescence, offer several advantages over home exercise programs. Experience in numerous cardiac exercise programs has demonstrated the value of medical or allied health personnel for exercise guidance, for motivation, and emergency care of exercise-related cardiovascular complications. The group exercise program, under medical supervision, also facilitates periodic or continuous ECG and blood pressure monitoring, particularly valuable in select patients.

Group programs offer advantages for patient teaching and instruction, promote compliance with the overall medical program, and permit validation of the exercise prescription and verification of the patient's ability to implement the exercise program safely and effectively. Finally, group programs may also serve to provide psychosocial support, promote understanding of the disease and its treatment, and reduce patient anxiety and depression.

Compliance is another issue when considering the recommendation of group versus home exercise programs. Many individuals prefer group over individual exercise. Social reinforcement through camaraderie and companionship of group programs may be motivators for exercise compliance.

COMMUNITY EXERCISE PROGRAMS (PHASE III)

Participants in community exercise programs may have progressed through hospital inpatient, and outpatient programs or may have been referred without previous participation. These programs may accept patients with various cardiorespiratory problems, depending on clinical judgment, facilities, equipment and availability of qualified staff. As a general rule, community based exercise programs include patients who are approximately 6 to 12 weeks after hospital discharge, have clinically stable or decreasing angina, medically controlled arrhythmias during exercise, a knowledge of symptoms, and the ability to self-regulate their exercise. Frequently, pulmonary patients and those with inadequately controlled hypertension may also benefit from such programs. Admission criteria vary and must be based on clinical and policy judgments. The community program provides an on-going maintenance program in which patients generally stay a minimum of 4 to 6 months. The suggested minimum functional capacity of participants in the community program is 5 METs but patients with a lower MET capacity may be admitted depending on local circumstances. Community programs are not generally located in clinical settings but may be offered three or more times per week in community facilities. An effective community program requires a minimum of two qualified staff members, (ACSM certified exercise specialists or Program Directors, for example) standing orders for emergency procedures, emergency equipment, and an on-call emergency team, and a staff-patient ratio of not greater than 1:10. All staff should be trained in CPR. Electrocardiographic monitoring can be performed in a community setting but this is not typical and requires additional staff and equipment.

Efforts should be made to move participants gradually to programs with less supervision. Participants who prove that they can self-regulate their exercise programs should be given increased freedom to do so. For patients with known cardiac disease the exercise test and medical evaluation should be continued on a 3 to 6 month basis and eventually on an annual basis or as needed.

EXERCISE PRESCRIPTION METHODS

Since most participants in community exercise programs have functional capacities greater than 5 METs, the exercise prescription methods described in Chapter 3 are usually applicable. During the first 3 to 6 months of participation the patient's exercise prescription should be gradually increased up to a duration 45 minutes or more of exercise at 50 to 85% of functional capacity, 3 to 4 sessions per week. After the desired functional capacity has been attained (usually 8 METs or more), maintenance should be the principal goal of the community exercise program.

Primary concerns of community programs should be promotion of compliance with the exercise prescription and other behavior modification goals. Since the ultimate goal for patients is lifelong adherence to exercise and because patients often remain in community programs for many months, special attention must be paid to patient motivation. It is, therefore, recommended that community programs include various exercise modalities and supplement the formal exercise prescription with low to moderate intensity recreational activities.

CRITERIA FOR DISCHARGE FROM A COMMUNITY PROGRAM

The duration of a community program varies depending upon local program guidelines but most programs start between 6 and 12 weeks after hospital discharge and last between 6 and 12 months. These programs may or may not be preceeded by an outpatient program. Standard criteria for discharge from a community program lack universal agreement and are not currently defined, nevertheless, suggested criteria are similar to those proposed for discharge from an outpatient program as outlined above.

Functional Capacity. After 3 to 12 months of participation in a community program a higher functional capacity can be expected. Since most vocational and recreational activities have a wide variance, the expected functional capacity should be related to the vocational and recreational demands which are pertinent to a given individual. A careful interview should yield the necessary information for making this decision on an individual basis. At the very least, a 5 MET capacity would allow a safe range of metabolic reserve for most of the necessary daily activities.

Medical Status. The same criteria established above for the patient being discharged from a Phase II program can be applied here.

Physical Fitness. The criteria for discharge of a Phase II patient apply here as well. It should be anticipated that the patient who has participated in an extended community program will have a greater functional reserve, and will be more likely to be interested in activities with a higher metabolic demand.

Education. The criteria outlined for the educational characteristics of the patient being discharged from a Phase II program can also be used for the Phase III patient. However, it should be emphasized that the Phase III patients will have participated for a greater length of time and presumably will have received more frequent evaluation in order to monitor progress and provide feedback. Specific mechanisms of follow-up evaluation need to be incorporated in order to modify the intervention plan if necessary and ensure that the educational objectives are being met.

SPECIAL CONSIDERATIONS

ANGINA PECTORIS

Patients with stable angina are excellent candidates for exercise programs. The object of physical conditioning in the patient with angina is to increase the amount of exercise performed before the onset of limiting angina. The patient must be evaluated for ischemic responses before, during, and after the exercise test. An essential element of this evaluation is the patient's description of the anginal episodes. This evaluation should include: (a) verbal description of symptoms (e.g., discomfort, pressure, tightness, burning, shortness of breath); (b) location of symptoms (e.g., substernal, jaw, teeth, throat, interscapular area, elbow, arm, wrist, epigastrium); (c) observed actions of the patient (e.g., clenched fist, rubbing); (d) duration and frequency of the episodes; (e) precipitating factors (e.g., rest, exertion, emotion); and (f) methods used to relieve the angina (e.g., rest, nitroglycerin). In evaluating the angina patient, consideration should be given to severity of disease, masking of symptoms by medications and abnormal blood pressure responses in exercise. Palpation of the painful chest area may help in differentiating musculoskeletal chest pain from that of the true angina. Teaching the patient to grade the angina symptom during the exercise test may be beneficial in determining the intensity of the discomfort for test termination (+3) and to judge exertion end points (+2) during an exercise session.

Many patients with angina experience the onset of symptoms at low levels of exercise, i.e., 2 to 3 METs. Exercise test protocols beginning at 1.5 to 2 METs help to identify onset of angina for these patients. Medication or exercise conditioning may produce subtle changes in MET capacity, heart rate, and blood pressure responses of patients with angina. Exercise test protocols of 0.5 MET increments may reflect these changes. Initial testing without drugs is helpful in estimating the magnitude of the ischemic response, however, patients on antianginal medications whose functional capacity is being evaluated for exercise prescription should continue medications as usual prior to testing. Administration of nitrates before or during the exercise test may add information for the exercise prescription. If beta blocking or calcium channel blocking medications are prescribed following evaluation of the diagnostic test, the exercise test should be repeated when the maintenance dosage is achieved. This reevaluation will establish the patient's medicated response during exercise and allow a more accurate exercise prescription.

Exercise intensity for angina patients should be set just below the anginal threshold. This intensity combined with the frequency and duration as described in Chapter 3 should elicit the desired conditioning responses. The exact exercise intensity may be determined by whether the patient is participating in a supervised or unsupervised program. The expected ischemic, arrhythmic, and anginal responses at specific conditioning intensities should be noted in the exercise prescription.

For the patient with angina, the exercise session should begin with a prolonged warm-up of at least 10 minutes' duration. After the warm-up, the aerobic phase of the exercise session can begin. Patients with angina may benefit from intermittent exercise in which exercise at prescribed intensities is followed by rest periods. This arrangement may be continued until the patient with angina has sufficient strength and stamina to sustain continuous exercise. Efforts should be made to utilize all major muscle groups, including the upper extremities. It is especially important to emphasize dynamic repetitive motions and to eliminate any tendency toward breath-holding. Patients should be cautioned not to exercise through angina when the discomfort continues to increase beyond a +2 intensity level. Rather, the patient should decrease activity until the discomfort subsides before continuing exercise at the previous intensity. Cool-down should be gradual and prolonged, at least 10 minutes, to prevent complications created by hydrostatic blood pooling in the lower extremities. Caution should be used when supervising patients for whom prophylactic use of nitroglycerin or long acting nitrates has been prescribed before or during exercise (e.g., blood pressure should be checked prior to use of nitroglycerin). Adverse hypotensive responses may occur in these patients, especially if they are taking other medications which may cause a decrease in blood pressure, (e.g., antiarrhythmics, beta blockers (propranolol), diuretics (hydrochlorothiazide)). If exertional angina is not relieved by terminating exercise or by the use of 3 sublingual nitroglycerin tablets (1 taken every 5 minutes), the patient should be transported to the nearest hospital emergency room.

PATIENTS WITH PACEMAKERS

Pacemakers are implanted to help manage conduction or rhythm disturbances which may occur with or without other forms of cardiac malfunction. Exercise prescription for patients with pacemakers requires knowledge of individual heart rate, blood pressure, and symptom response to exercise; and an understanding of the underlying conduction abnormality, pacemaker type and programming, and left ventricular function.

The two major conditions leading to pacemaker implantation are sick sinus syndrome (SSS) and high degree AV node block (AVB). SSS and AVB may coexist and either may show intermittent or fixed abnormalities. SSS is characterized by episodes of bradycardia (sinus bradycardia or sinus pauses), sometimes episodic atrial tachyarrhythmias (fibrillation flutter) and often by chronotropic insufficiency. AVB is most commonly manifest as complete heart block (atria beating independently of an idioventricular rhythm which is usually at a fixed slow rate).

A pacing system consists of a generator and one or two leads. The leads are commonly placed via a central vein, and may be positioned in the right ventricular apex (single chamber pacer), right atrium and right ventricle (dual-chamber), or rarely in the right atrium alone. Leads can be positioned on the epicardium surgically, but this is rarely done in adults. The leads conduct impulses from the generator to the heart (resulting in stimulation) and from the heart to the generator (allowing the generator to "sense" intrinsic cardiac activity). Many parameters of generator function, such as minimum rate, level of sensitivity to intrinsic cardiac activity and output may be changed noninvasively after implantation using a programmer. Most implanted generators have functions which are programmable.

Since pacemakers may sense and pace in the ventricle, atrium, or both, and may respond to sensed intrinsic events by being inhibited or by firing (stimulating), a three position code has been developed to describe individual pacemaker function. The first position describes the chamber(s) paced, the second describes the chamber(s) sensed, and the third the mode of response. The most commonly implanted pacing system has a single lead which paces only the right *V*entricle, senses only the right *V*entricle, and responds to sensed activity by *I*nhibiting generator output. This is described as a VVI (a "demand" ventricular pacemaker). A pacemaker with leads in the atrium and ventricle (*D*ual-chambered), which paces *D*ual-chamber, can sense *D*ual-chamber and may inhibit or stimulate is designated DDD. Many other varieties of response and derived codes exist and a single generator may be programmed to various modes.

The specific problem posed by pacemakers during exercise is the rate-response to increased activity. The most commonly used pacing system (VVI) cannot stimulate the heart faster than its programmed rate (often 70 bpm). If AV node conduction is absent, ventricular rate remains constant even if the atrial rate rises with exercise. Thus the main cardiac response to demand for higher cardiac output is lost in patients with AVB. If AV conduction is intact, as it may in patients with SSS or intermittent AVB, ventricular rate may rise with atrial rate.

Dual-chamber pacemakers solve this problem for many patients. If atrial rate rises with exercise, the atrial lead senses this and the generator stimulates the ventricles at this increased rate, thus restoring rate responsiveness and its contribution to a rise in cardiac output. However, the rise in atrial rate on which this depends may be limited by medication (beta-blockers, digitalis) or by such conditions as SSS.

In patients with an abnormal rate-response to exercise (absent or blunted), cardiac output can rise primarily by increasing stroke volume. The magnitude of this change is limited by abnormalities in left ventricular function. Prior to performing exercise treadmill tests and prescribing exercise for such patients, clinical data should be reviewed regarding the status of left ventricular fuction and the presence or absence of coexisting valvular, congenital, or coronary artery disease. In performing exercise treadmill tests, close attention must be paid to symptoms, RPE, and blood pressure response.

Exercise prescriptions for these patients should be based on the treadmill test and closely monitored, paying careful attention to resting and exercise blood pressure measurement, RPE, and symptom development. Patients with pacemakers can engage in most training activities appropriate for their functional capacity and underlying heart disease, but some physicians may prefer avoidance of excessive upper extremity and shoulder motion. A properly functioning pacemaker protects against slow rates but unless it has special antitachycardia functions, ventricular tachyarrhythmias may occur and require the same management as in non-paced patients with heart disease.

Development of the exercise prescription for the heart rate responsive pacemaker patient may be developed in a similar manner as previously described for patients with coronary heart disease. Proper attention must be paid to the underlying cardiac abnormality that necessitated the pacemaker as noted above. Patients with congenital or valvular heart disease may require modification of their individual exercise prescription based upon their physiologic and functional limitations.

In developing the exercise prescription for patients with fixed heart rates the standard ACSM guidelines for TYPE, DURATION, and FREQUENCY of exercise should be employed. However, intensity of exercise should be prescribed on the basis of blood pressure response to the exercise test. Additional cardiovascular warm-up and avoidance of torso bending exercises are suggested with added emphasis on a gradual return of the vascular state to its normal resting status. Assessment of systolic blood pressure at least 3 times during training sessions is suggested until the subject is familiar and comfortable with his/her individual response to exercise training. Measurement of resting blood pressure is often helpful if the presence of exercise associated hypotension is to be assessed during the exercise session.

The intensity portion of the exercise prescription for patients with fixed heart rates can be developed by employing a modified Karvonen equation applied to the systolic blood pressure.

Standard Karvonen Equation

$$\text{THR} = (\text{HR}_{max} - \text{HR}_{rest})(0.6 \text{ to } 0.8) + \text{HR}_{rest}$$

Modified Karvonen Equation

$$\text{TSBP} = (\text{SBP}_{max} - \text{SBP}_{rest})(0.6 \text{ to } 0.8) + \text{SBP}_{rest}$$

THR = Training Heart Rate
TSBP = Training Systolic Blood Pressure

Precautions

Special precautions in this unique population include:

- Exercise precautions based upon the underlying cardiac abnormality are of the utmost importance.

- If the patient has had a long-standing need for pacemaker support, and may have received the pacemaker recently, the previous relatively sedentary lifestyle may have resulted in a severe deconditioned state.
- Battery and pacemaker function should be assessed at appropriate intervals.
- The placement of a pacemaker for electrical instability does not eliminate the need for arrythmia precautions.
- Blood pressure may not respond to physical activity in the manner expected in a non-paced patient. This is especially important in patients with fixed rate pacemakers. Appropriate attention must be given to warmup, cooldown and exercise tolerance.
- Over prolonged periods electrodes tend to become relatively fixed. Nonetheless, caution is advised regarding excessive stretching and body manipulation.

CARDIAC MEDICATIONS

Drug therapy is an important component of the overall program of medical care for many cardiac patients. Many of the medications that are commonly prescribed for cardiac patients may impact on cardiorespiratory and/or metabolic responses to exercise. Thus it is important that, in developing exercise prescriptions for cardiac patients, the effect of drug regimens be considered. The expected physiologic effects of the common cardiac medications are summarized in Appendix B.

In general, it is recommended that the cardiac patient's exercise prescription be based on responses to an exercise test administered while following the patient's normal drug regimen. In the early post-discharge phase of exercise rehabilitation, patients may frequently have their drug regimen changed. It is imperative that the exercise leader be informed of these changes, and alterations in the exercise prescription may be necessary. In some cases, re-administration of an exercise test may be helpful.

Medications used in the management of heart disease affect exercise performance both by their intrinsic effects and by modification of the pathophysiologic conditions for which they are used.

The effects of a consistent drug regimen on exercise are demonstrated by exercise testing, but changes in dose, addition or deletion of medications, or variations in patient adherence may lead to problems in exercise prescription. Thus patients in exercise programs must be repeatedly instructed to report changes in treatment. Generally, it is impractical to repeat exercise treadmill tests after each change in drug therapy.

Among cardiac drugs, beta blockers have the greatest effect on exercise prescription. Calcium channel blockers, nitrates and other vasodilators may alter heart rate, blood pressure and angina threshold. Digitalis and anti-arrhythmics have little effect on exercise prescription.

Beta Blockers

Beta blockers were originally used in cardiac populations in the management of angina and arrhythmias (atrial or ventricular). More recently, several studies have demonstrated a reduction in mortality in patients given these agents following recovery from myocardial infarction. Thus they are used frequently and personnel involved in exercise programs for cardiac patients need a knowledge of the various agents and their effects on exercise prescription.

Beta blockers lower resting heart rate, blood pressure, and exercise heart rate at any given exercise intensity. In patients with exertional angina, beta blockers usually allow a higher achieved workload through their effect of lowering heart rate and blood pressure (and thus myocardial oxygen demand); the anginal threshold is raised. If used in patients with severe left ventricular dysfunction, beta blockers may substantially lower achieved workload through their negative inotropic effects. In subjects without angina or mild left ventricular dysfunction beta blockers may lower maximal workload. Resting and exercise-induced fatigue may occur, especially with non-selective beta blocker use.

Beta blocker use changes significantly the relationships among heart rate, perceived exertion, and exercise intensity. Although any of these parameters can be used for exercise prescription, close attention must be paid to MET equivalents, which are particularly useful in adjusting a training program if drug dose is altered.

Calcium Channel Blockers (Calcium Antagonists)

Currently marketed calcium antagonists include nifedipine, verapamil, diltiazem. These agents block calcium-dependent contraction in vascular smooth muscle and myocardial cells. They thus act as coronary and peripheral vasodilators and have variable negative inotropic effects. In addition, verapamil in particular is used in the management of supraventricular tachycardia. Any of these agents may lead to variable degrees of AV block in susceptible patients.

Calcium antagonists are used primarily as antianginal agents. In patients limited by angina, calcium antagonists may increase exercise capacity by mechanisms described above. In patients without angina, little effect on peak exercise intensity would be expected. Because of peripheral vasodilatation, nifedipine in particular sometimes causes resting tachycardia. Conversely, verapamil may lower resting heart rate. As with beta blockers, the agent and dose used must be noted at the time of exercise testing and changes in rest and exercise heart rate should be anticipated if medication changes occur.

Antiarrhythmic Agents

Although not much information is available regarding the specific effects of antiarrhythmic agents on exercise testing, prescription or training, little effect is expected. It is important to know that in addition to their antidysrhythmic effects, any of these agents may in some conditions worsen the dysrhythmia for which they are being used. Exercise heart rate should be monitored frequently in such patients, especially if medication changes are made. In addition, substantial day-to-day and hour-to-hour variability exists in PVC frequency and complexity. Thus rhythm disturbances seen on exercise testing may bear a variable relationship to those seen during exercise training.

Nitrates

The most frequently encountered nitrate preparations include short acting sublingual nitroglycerin, nitroglycerin ointment or discs, and long-acting nitrates. These agents act as coronary artery vasodilators, but their principal antianginal effect is probably a result of venous dilitation which reduces cardiac preload and thus myocardial oxygen consumption. Nitrates may alter exercise capacity in patients limited by angina by increasing the anginal threshold. In patients who develop exertional angina, sublingual nitroglycerin will potentiate exercise-induced venous dilitation and may result in hypotension. Such patients should cool down slowly following exercise testing or training session.

REFERENCES

Amsterdam EA, Wilmore JH and Demaria AN: *Exercise in Cardiovascular Health and Disease.* New York: Yorke Medical Books, 1977.

Committee on Exercise. *Exercise testing and training of individuals with heart disease or at high risk for its development.* Dallas: American Heart Association, 1975.

Oldridge WB, Wicks JR, Hanley C, Sutton JR and Jones NL: Non-compliance in an exercise rehabilitation program for men who have suffered a myocardial infarction. *Can Med Assoc J, 118*:361–364, 1978.

Pollock ML, Ward A and Foster C: Exercise prescription for rehabilitation of the cardiac patient. In: Pollock ML and Schmidt DH. *Heart Disease and Rehabilitation.* Boston: Houghton Mifflin, 1979.

Superko HR: The effects of cardiac rehabilitation in permanently paced patients with third degree heart block. *J Cardiac Rehabil, 3*:561–568, 1983.

5

Exercise Prescription for Special Populations

The process of exercise prescription involves developing a balanced program which has the potential for improving the functional capacity and health status of specific individuals. When an individual has identified medical problems or diagnosed disease, the exercise prescription must be modified to enable the participant with special circumstances to make the best physiologic and psychologic adjustment to the conditioning program.

In this chapter guidelines are presented for prescription of exercise in patients who manifest selected diseases and clinical conditions.

PULMONARY DISEASE

Exercise training is an important aspect of rehabilitation of patients with chronic obstructive pulmonary disease (COPD). Although it has been demonstrated that aerobic exercise fails to improve indices of pulmonary function (lung volume, airway resistance, arterial blood gases, etc.), exercise may improve cardiovascular function, muscular strength and endurance and physiologic capacity in COPD patients. Exercise training also has been reported to increase the patient's social activity, improve the patient's ability to tolerate activities of daily living, decrease fear of exercise, increase tolerance of dyspnea, improve sleep and appetite, decrease anxiety and promote adjustment to disability.

Patients with pulmonary disease should be clinically assessed by a pulmonologist. Exercise test protocols may be continuous or discontinuous due to the limited functional capacity often associated with pulmonary disease. Small increases in exercise intensity are recommended. The patient is likely to achieve a higher maximal exercise level if the time spent at each test stage is short. The most common reason patients give for stopping the test is dyspnea. Essential variables to be measured during the graded exercise test, in addition to ECG and blood pressure, include ventilation, respiratory frequency, and tidal volume. Other important information may be obtained from oxygen uptake, carbon dioxide output, and non-invasive measurement of the arterial oxygen saturation (SaO_2). Arterial blood gas analysis may be important in patients with gas exchange disturbances.

The exercise prescription must be individualized in accordance with the patient's degree of respiratory disability. Ideally the exercise prescription should be determined in consultation with the referring physician, and should take into account the degree of respiratory disability as assessed clinically, through pulmonary function tests.

Patients with essentially normal spirometry who experience dyspnea only on heavy exercise respond to exercise training much as do patients with cardiovascular disease and the heart rate method may be used to designate exercise intensity as described elsewhere in this book. When the forced vital capacity (FVC) and FEV_1 are between 60 to 80% of predicted, patients may experience dyspnea when walking rapidly. Reductions in ventilatory capacity usually are not the limiting factor to exercise in these patients. Generally, exercise intensity should be maintained at the level that requires ventilatory rate less than 75% of the patient's maximal exercise ventilation.

More severely limited patients (FVC and $FEV_1 < 60\%$ of predicted, abnormal V_D/V_T at rest and/or exercise with or without desaturation during exercise) who experience difficulty breathing with only mild exercise are limited by their respiratory system. Patients who exhibit an abnormal breathing pattern during the exercise test may be helped by advice regarding proper breathing techniques. Some severely limited patients may require supplemental oxygen during the activity if this has been objectively demonstrated to improve exercise performance. During exercise testing it is recommended that supplemental oxygen be administered through a high flow O_2 enrichment system giving an inspired O_2 concentration of 24 or 28%.

The assistance of a respiratory therapist may be valuable in this regard.

Modifications in the duration and frequency of exercise may be required. For example, pulmonary patients may benefit from two 10-minute sessions or even four 5-minute sessions daily. As an individual's tolerance to exercise improves, the duration or intensity of each session may progressively increase. The type of exercise is essentially the same as for cardiac patients. Brisk walking, jogging, and cycling are useful activities. Swimming techniques, modified by the use of swim fins and a kickboard, also may be useful. Upper body aerobic exercise, such as rowing and arm cranking are generally not applicable because of the high ventilation required at a given power output in this type of exercise. The mode of exercise should be something which the patient is interested in and preferably an exercise which will directly improve the patient's ability to do usual daily activities. Ventilatory muscle training either by breathing against an inspiratory resistance or by isocapnic hyperpnea may improve respiratory muscle strength and endurance and consequently exercise capacity. Experience with this modality, however, is limited and its role in the exercise program is not yet firmly established.

DIABETES MELLITUS

In prescribing exercise for diabetics it is important to distinguish between the two types of diabetes. Type I diabetes (previously called insulin dependent or juvenile diabetes) results from a pancreatic deficiency in insulin production. The Type I diabetic is dependent on regular administration of exogenous insulin. Type II diabetes (previously called non insulin dependent or maturity onset diabetes) is usually associated with excessive concentrations of insulin, decreased cellular insulin sensitivity and obesity. This form of diabetes is typically treated with dietary modification, exercise and medications (e.g., oral hypoglycemics). Although not always necessary insulin is often administered to the Type II diabetics.

Several general factors should be considered in developing an exercise prescription for the diabetic. An exercise program is not recommended for uncontrolled diabetics. Two potential problems occur in exercising insulin-medicated diabetics. The first problem is that lack of sufficient insulin may cause a hyperglycemic effect in the blood because cellular absorption of glucose is restricted. A second problem is the hypoglycemic effect which occurs due to an increased mobilization of depot insulin, particularly if the injection site was in the exercising muscle. Since physical activity has an insulin-like effect, the exercise program requires an insulin dependent diabetic to either reduce insulin intake or increase carbohydrate intake. It is important to instruct the diabetic participant and the exercise staff that during prolonged activities adequate nourishment must be available in the form of sugar, fruit juice, and/or other readily digestible carbohydrates. The exercise program director and the exercise specialist should be aware of any participants who are diabetic and their hypoglycemic symptoms. Special attention should be paid to patients taking insulin and beta blocker medication because the hypoglycemic symptoms may be masked by the beta blocker.

Since exercise may precipitate a hypoglycemic event in diabetics (particularly Type I), it is recommended that the diabetic exercise with a partner, be knowledgeable of the signs and symptoms of hypoglycemia and carry a carbohydrate source during exercise. Generally diabetics can avoid hypoglycemic events by:

1. monitoring blood glucose more frequently when initiating an exercise program,
2. decreasing the insulin dose (1 to 2 units or as recommended by the physician) or increasing carbohydrate intake (10 to 15 grams per one-half hour of exercise) prior to an exercise bout,
3. injecting insulin in an area such as the abdomen that will not be active during exercise,
4. avoiding exercise during periods of peak insulin activity, and
5. eating carbohydrate snacks before and during prolonged exercise bouts.

Longterm elevation of blood glucose may lead to microangiopathy and neuropathy. This may lead to impairment of peripheral circulation and anhidrosis (i.e., failure of the sweat mechanism). Consequently diabetic exercisers should take particular care in selecting footwear, should practice good foot hygiene and should be particularly cautious when exercising in conditions of heat stress.

In general, diabetics can participate in the same modes of activity as non-diabetics. However, for the obese diabetic non-weight bearing activities minimize risk of orthopedic injury. The frequency of exercise should be 5 to 7 days per week for both types of diabetics. For the Type I diabetic, exercise should be performed daily so that a regular pattern of diet and insulin dosage can be maintained. The Type II diabetic should exercise at least 5 days per week to maximize caloric expenditure for the purpose of weight management.

The recommended duration of exercise is specific to the type of diabetes. Because the Type I diabetic's frequency of exercise is high, duration can be as low as 20 to 30 minutes per exercise. In contrast, with Type II diabetics the emphasis should be on maximizing caloric expenditure and duration as long as 40 to 60 minutes per session are recommended.

Intensity of exercise for the diabetic should be prescribed within the normal range (50 to 85% of functional capacity). However, it is recommended that Type I diabetics avoid or be carefully monitored during high intensity exercise of long duration since this type of activity may lead to hypoglycemic reactions. Episodes of hypoglycemia may occur as late as 24 to 48 hours following an exercise session and patients should be made aware of this possibility. In Type II diabetics, because frequency and duration of exercise are high, intensity should be maintained near the lower end (50 to 65%) of the functional capacity range. For most diabetics exercise intensity can be prescribed by the heart rate method. However, the diabetic with autonomic neuropathy demonstrates chronotropic insufficiency during exercise. Therefore, the perceived exertion or MET methods may be preferred in regulating exercise intensity in patients with neuropathy. Patients with advanced retinopathy should not perform activities which cause excessive jarring or marked increases in blood pressure. Swimming is a recommended activity for patients with retinopathy.

OBESITY

An exercise program for the obese patient should be one component of a comprehensive weight management program which may include restriction of caloric intake, medications, surgical procedure, and/or behavior modification. The obese patient presents special problems related to exercise testing and prescription. If walking on the motor driven treadmill is not possible, a cycle ergometer should be used to test functional capacity. Obese patients are prone to conditions of syncope during an exercise session. This response occurs due to fluid imbalance resulting from restriction of caloric intake and exercise induced fluid loss. Syncope can be alleviated by having the patient assume the hook lying position during the cool-down phase of the exercise session.

The exercise prescription for the obese patient should emphasize caloric expenditure. Bicycle and other weight supported activities are recommended since they minimize risk of orthopedic problems. *Intensity* should be prescribed at approximately 50% of functional capacity and *duration* should be adjusted based on body weight to elicit a caloric deficit of approximately 1750 calories (0.25 kg) per week. Combined weight loss through diet and exercise should not exceed 1 kg per week. *Frequency* of exercise should be designed to distribute the total caloric expenditure throughout the week with a duration for each session that can be well tolerated. A frequency of 3 per week would require a 600 calorie expenditure each session. For some patients, it may be more appropriate to increase the frequency to 5 per week and reduce the duration to elicit a calorie expenditure of 350 calories per session. As fitness level increases and body weight decreases the exercise prescription should be modified to maintain the desired caloric expenditure.

In addition to a specified exercise program, obese patients should be encouraged to modify their exercise behaviors throughout the daily routine to further increase caloric expenditure. This can be accomplished by increasing body movement during work, social activity, and recreational pursuits.

Patient education is an important component of the weight management program. Long term adherence and subsequent permanent life style changes relative to diet and exercise requires an appreciation and understanding of the following effects of exercise: (1) exercise promotes negative energy balance during the exercise session, (2) exercise increases metabolic rate for an extended period of time following the session, (3) exercise may counteract the decrease in metabolic rate associated with hypocaloric diet, (4) exercise may have a short term effect of suppressing appetite, and (5) exercise is a good alternative activity to eating, which is often a response to stress in obese individuals.

HYPERTENSION

Exercise guidelines and prescription must be adjusted to accomodate a multitude of situations. The mode of exercise and the effect of various hypertensive agents on exercise performance are important considerations for the selection of activities of patients with high blood pressure.

Mean arterial pressure increases during dynamic and isometric exercise; however, dynamic exercise is associated with a rise of systolic blood pressure while isometric exercise is associated predominantly with an increase of diastolic blood pressure. High anaerobic work also elicits a pressor response. Thus isometric and high intensity exercise are not recommended for patients with high blood pressure.

An increasing proportion of patients with essential hypertension are controlling their blood pressure with effective and well-tolerated antihypertensive agents. However, these medications may modify the acute or chronic physiologic response to exercise. Thus, to properly prescribe exercise as therapy, it is important to be familiar with the physiologic alterations produced by various pharmacologic agents encountered in dealing with patients with essential hypertension.

Diuretics. Diuretic therapy is often encountered in patients with mild to moderate hypertension. Diuretics prevent the reabsorption of electrolytes and water at various sites in the renal tubules. Under normal circumstances, diuretics do not alter resting or maximal heart rate, exercise performance or exercise capacity. Thus training heart rate should be determined in the standard way. However, patients may experience a diuretic-induced hypokalemia, which combined with exercise can precipitate dangerous arrhythmias. Combination of diuretic therapy and exercise may also produce rhabdomyolysis, secondary aldosteronemia, and hyperuricemia. Potassium sparing diuretics are often helpful in maintaining potassium balance and in preventing these anomalies.

Beta Blockers. The blood pressure lowering effect of beta blockers has been attributed to a reduction of cardiac output, suppression of renin, interference with central sympathetic outflow, and prevention of neurotransmitter release by stimulation of presynaptic receptors. Beta blockade produces a reduction of heart rate and cardiac output at rest and during submaximal and maximal exercise. These hemodynamic alterations may be dose dependent. Exercise training intensity based on heart rate must be adjusted to a percentage of the maximal heart rate attained while on beta blockade therapy. Exercise and beta blockade may induce hyperkalemia.

Vasodilators. Vasodilators relax the smooth muscle of arterioles or veins. Vasodilators may cause a reflex tachycardia that may accelerate symptoms of angina. It is important that patients on vasodilators cool down adequately following an exercise session to prevent hypotension. Since vasodilators do not alter heart rate response to increasing workloads, exercise intensity can be based on heart rate using standard procedures.

Angiotensin Converting Enzyme Inhibitor. These drugs inhibit the enzyme activity that converts angiotensin I to the potent vasoconstrictor angiotensin II. Since these drugs do not affect hemodynamic or heart rate response to exercise, exercise intensity may be prescribed in the standard manner.

Calcium Channel Blocking Agents. These medications inhibit the calcium influx into cardiac and vascular smooth muscle cells. Calcium channel blockers may alter heart rate and hemodynamic variables at rest and during exercise (the effects may be different with different drugs) and therefore the exercise prescription should be based on the medicated patient's individual response to an exercise test.

CNS Active. These agents act as false neurotransmitters, central alpha agonists or depletors of neuronal stores of catecholamines within the central nervous system. The several specific medications in this category have varying effects on heart rate and hemodynamic variables during exercise. As such, the exercise prescription should be developed with caution. In particular, it should be noted that exercise may produce hypotension, dizziness and syncope in patients taking several of the central antagonists (e.g., Ismelin, Serpasil, Serapres).

Alpha Blocker. These drugs cause relaxation of peripheral arterioles via blockade of postsynaptic alpha-adrenoreceptors. Alpha blockers lower exercise diastolic and systolic blood pressures but do not affect the heart rate response to exercise. Therefore, heart rate methods for prescribing exercise intensity may be used in the normal manner.

PERIPHERAL VASCULAR DISEASE

Individuals with significant peripheral vascular disease are at a much higher risk of having associated coronary and cerebral vascular disease than those without peripheral impairment. Intermittent testing protocols may be advantageous when evaluating these patients for exercise. Subjective gradation of pain is a useful technique for expressing claudication discomfort and can be divided into the following general categories:

Grade IV—Excrutiating and unbearable pain.

Grade III—Intense pain (short of Grade IV) from which the patient's attention cannot be diverted except by catastrophic events (i.e., fire, explosion).

Grade II—Moderate discomfort or pain from which the patient's attention can be diverted by a number of common stimuli (i.e., conversation, an interesting episode on T.V.).

Grade I—Definite discomfort or pain but only of initial or modest level (established—but minimal).

Activity should consist of daily aerobic activity (a minimum of 5 days a week), and preferably with two periods of exercise per day. Activities might include walking, stationary bicycling, swimming or pool activities where the patient is exercised in shallow warm water. Intensity of exercise must be balanced between the Grade II pain level and the prescribed target heart rate. The duration of each exercise session should be at least 20 minutes. Intermittent rest periods may be necessary.

ARTHRITIS

Exercise producing excess stress on osteoarthritic joints should be avoided. A specific exercise program should be performed daily to maintain and improve both range of joint motion and muscle strength. Exercises should not be severely painful, but slight pain may be tolerated. Exercise periods of short duration and increasing frequency impose less stress on osteoarthritic joints.

Patients who have rheumatoid arthritis are limited in their ability to adhere to a specific exercise regimen because of the complication arising from the arthritic problem. Weight bearing activities, for example, are contraindicated during inflammatory episodes in the lower extremities. However, every effort must be made to sustain satisfactory levels of muscular strength and range of motion.

For many patients with osteoarthritis or rheumatoid arthritis a walk-jog program might be stressful. Alternatives to the walk-jog exercise include cycling, arm-ergometry, and rowing. Swimming is often recommended as an acceptable exercise. The intensity of a swimming exercise prescription depends upon the patient's proficiency in the water, their ability to modify swimming strokes to minimize the stress to the affected joints, and their target heart rates.

MENTAL ILLNESS

Exercise training is sometimes employed in the treatment of mental illnesses such as depression. In general, the principles of exercise prescription discussed in Chapter 3 are appropriate for these patients. However, patients with mental illnesses often take prescribed drugs, some of which can alter the metabolic and cardiorespiratory responses to exercise.

Four classes of drugs are particularly likely to be used in patients with mental illness: Major tranquilizers (mainly phenothiazines), minor tranquilizers (e.g., diazepam), antidepressants (particularly tricyclics), and lithium carbonate. There is little known about the effects of these drugs on exercise, except as predicted from their general pharmacology. Phenothiazines have complex effects on the cardiovascular system, produced by alpha-adrenergic receptor blockade, direct myocardial depression, and other direct and indirect action. Electrocardiographic changes include T-wave, alterations, U-waves, and prolongation of the Q-T interval. Tricyclic antidepressants have anticholinergic effects, block uptake of catecholamines in cardiac adrenergic nerves, and have other cardiovascular effects. They have been associated with hypotension, congestive heart failure, myocardial infarction, and sudden death. Tricyclics increase the PR and Q-T intervals and produce T-wave change. Lithium carbonate produces prolonged Q-T intervals, T-wave inversion or flattening, and premature ventricular contractions. Lithium levels are affected by sodium metabolism which can be affected by exercise. Elevations in lithium have been associated with sudden death, seizures, and other side effects. The precise implication of these drug induced ECG changes on exercise and exercise testing is unclear, but may be important in interpretation of exercise test results. These drugs should be used with caution in patients with cardiovascular disease, and exercise effects should be carefully monitored.

PREGNANCY

Pregnancy, though not a disease, is a condition that involves special considerations in prescribing exercise. Contraindications for exercise during pregnancy include cardiovascular diseases, toxemia and eclampsia. Since the effects of exercise on pregnant women with hypertension, diabetes and obesity are unknown at this time, exercise should be used cautiously with these patients.

In selecting a mode of exercise pregnant women should avoid sporting activities that involve violent movements and/or physical contact. As body weight increases during the third trimester, a non-weight bearing activity should be employed. Intensity of exercise should be monitored near the low end of the normal prescriptive range to minimize oxygen debt and lactate production. Intensity and duration of exercise should be modified to avoid excessive increases in core temperature. The heart rate method for prescribing exercise intensity can be used. However, some evidence indicates that maximal heart rate may decline progressively during pregnancy. This may require reassessment and an adjustment of the target heart rate. Application of the RPE prescriptive technique may be appropriate.

The pregnant woman should make regular visits to her physician and should report any problems with her exercise.

RENAL DISEASE

Patients with end stage renal disease (ESRD) have three treatment options: hemodialysis (most common), peritoneal dialysis and transplantation. Exercise training may be especially beneficial for selected ESRD patients. Since hemodialysis is, at the present time, the most widely used treatment in the United States, the recommendations in this section pertain primarily to this group.

Hemodialysis patients typically utilize an artificial kidney machine 3 times per week for 4 to 5 hours per session. These patients experience dramatic fluid volume shifts, electrolyte abnormalities, hypertension and most are severely anemic. Over a long period of time they may develop cardiovascular complications due to the volume and pressure overload and many eventually develop congestive heart failure and/or accelerated atherosclerosis. Other problems common in this population include: renal osteodystrophy, muscle weakness and cramping, lipid abnormalities and abnormal psychologic profiles. Many hemodialysis patients are diabetic.

Most ESRD patients are extremely sedentary and exercise tolerance tends to be low (average 5 METS). Exercise training can increase exercise tolerance; improve blood pressure, muscle strength, and lipid profiles, and, in some patients, increase hematocrit. Patient selection is extremely important: only patients who are on a stable regimen of dialysis, diet and medication should be considered for an exercise program.

The exercise prescription must be low level, ideally beginning with non-weight bearing, interval activity (e.g. stationary cycling). Age predicted maximal heart rates are rarely, if ever achieved in dialysis patients. Therefore the rating of perceived exertion as a technique for designating exercise intensity is often the method of choice with ESRD patients. Exercise sessions should be monitored and adjustments should be made to accomodate the volume overloaded state, an increase in electrolytes (particularly potassium) or any other complications experienced by these patients. An 'off' dialysis day may be the best time for the exercise, however, compliance to such a program may be a problem. Cycle ergometry during hemodialysis treatment may offer the best promise for optimal compliance and supervision for these patients, however, the physiologic effects of such a program are not yet fully documented.

REFERENCES

Goldberg, AP, Geltman, EM, Hagberg, JM et al.: Therapeutic Benefits of Exercise Training for Hemodialysis Patients. Kidney Inter. *24*: Suppl. 16, S-303, 1983.

Leon AS, Conrad J, Hunninghake DB and Serfass R: Effects of a vigorous walking program on body composition and carbohydrate and lipid metabolism of obese young men. *Am J Clin Nutri, 33*:1776–1787, 1979.

Richter EA, Ruderman NB and Schneider SH: Diabetes and exercise. *Am J Med, 70*:201–209, 1981.

Unger KM, Moser KM, and Hansen P: Selection of an exercise program for patients with chronic obstructive pulmonary disease. *Heart Lung, 9*:68–76, 1980.

Zabetakis PM, Gleim GW, Pasternak FL, Saraniti A, Nicholas JA and Michelis MF: Long-duration submaximal exercise conditioning in hemodialysis patients. *Clin Nephrology, 18*:17, 1982.

6

Behavior Change

Exercise programs provide an opportunity for positively affecting a variety of health behaviors. The health fitness instructor, exercise test technologist, exercise specialist, health fitness director, and program director should be familiar with basic principles of behavior change and when appropriate use these techniques to help motivate clients to begin and maintain a healthy lifestyle. The intention or motivation to initiate a health behavior change, such as an exercise program, is influenced by somewhat different factors than those that maintain the behavior change.

The intention (or motivation) to initiate a healthy behavior is influenced by various factors such as:

1. perceived benefits of making the change,
2. perceived ease or difficulty of making the change,
3. information about the need to make the change,
4. models among family, friends, peers as well as print and electronic media,
5. previous experience,
6. incentives such as financial reward, improved well-being and health, and
7. disincentives such as cost and inconvenience.

The motivation to make positive behavior changes is optimized when the above factors are presented with role models of others benefiting, clear instructions, and information about the benefit. The review of success or failure with intended change may povide clues to successful individualization of the behavior change strategies. The change should be rewarding and achievable; confidence in being able to make change is increased by appropriate strategies such as small steps and gradual acquisition of new skills.

Once a behavior has been adopted, maintaining it is influenced by different factors. The physiologic and psychologic benefits a person receives from a health behavior change is a major factor influencing maintenance of behavior. Adherence (compliance) to newly established health behaviors is often threatened by changes such as vacations, illness or new schedules. Participants should make plans for how and when they will resume an exercise program following such disruptions.

Effective communication is critical to successfully motivate a person to initiate or maintain a health behavior program. An effective counselor primarily uses open-ended questions (rather than those answered by yes or no), allows the client to talk, tolerates periods of silence, and shows a non-judgmental, non-critical attitude toward lifestyle. The counselor should act as a facilitator, and not assume responsibility for the change or become too ego involved in the participant's eventual success or failure.

Other factors which are important for maintaining behavior change involve verbal and written feedback of progress, and continued individual and environmental incentives. For instance, feedback of improvement of functional capacity helps maintain a participant's interest in exercising. Emotional support from a spouse, institution or other community resource can also be helpful for maintaining behavioral change.

The exercise leader should be familiar with symptoms of major psychopathologic conditions which might interfere with a patient's ability to engage in health behavior change. Major mood disturbances such as depression might interfere with a patient's adherence to an exercise or other health behavior change program. The exercise leader should be alert for symptoms such as depressed mood or sexual desire, sleep disturbance (particularly early morning waking), loss of appetite, loss of interest in usual activities, sense of helplessness (including thoughts of suicide), and excess fatigue, which might indicate significant depression or other problems. Participants experiencing these (and other unusual symptoms) should be considered for referral and professional counseling. Problems with learning and retention also need special consideration.

Crises, like loss of a loved one or a major financial setback, can interrupt a participant's exercise program. People in crises often exhibit a major change in affect (like easy tearfulness) or behavior, become withdrawn or emotionally distant, or at times display inappropriate behavior. The exercise leader can play an important role in managing such crises by asking if the participant is having a problem, privately discussing the problem and suggesting referral to a specialist if appropriate. If they have stopped exercising, the participants should be encouraged to resume exercise when the crisis is resolved.

Some specific strategies which should be adopted for changing the various lifestyle factors related to health are described below.

ADHERENCE (COMPLIANCE) TO EXERCISE

Adherence to an exercise program is often poor. There is no single or simple technique to improve adherence in a large percentage of people. Factors which have been shown to reduce adherence to exercise are: orthopedic injuries, inadequate social support, personal and family problems, blue collar work, transportation difficulties, high perceived exertion, inconvenience, and expense. Smokers and overweight people have demonstrated poor adherence. Such factors should be taken into consideration in developing a program for an individual. Steps to help improve adherence to an exercise program include: (1) Evaluate the participants expectations for the exercise program. Are they realistic? How will the participants know when they have achieved their goal? (2) Determine what problems the participants anticipate. Why have they stopped exercising in the past? Employ problem solving techniques to achieve solutions to such anticipated disruptions. (3) Establish a method of determining the participant's adherence, such as program attendance, exercise logs, or periodic recall of exercise. (4) Employ problem solving techniques to achieve solutions to low adherence. What incentives or disincentives can be used to improve adherence? Phone-call prompts for attending programs, self-contracting, and regular monitoring by the participant and the counselor may also help improve adherence.

Some clients with low adherence may consume an inappropriate amount of staff time. Termination from a program should be considered when a participant is chronically absent or interruptive to a program. An agreement should be made with the participant specifying the level or duration of attendance or improvement in behavior expected for continuing in the program.

SMOKING

The exercise leader can play an important role in helping smokers quit. Particularly after they have established rapport with a client and in the context of showing concern, the exercise leader should ask if the participants want to quit and encourage them to do so. The following considerations may be useful in providing assistance.

1. Provide information on the dangers of smoking and the benefits of quitting. The connections between smoking and symptoms they have reported or are having, medical findings or other relevant concerns should be detailed. Emphasize that quitting smoking is probably the single most important action they can take to improve their health.
2. Determine the participant's willingness to quit.
3. Evaluate past failures and develop new strategies.
4. Request a quit date and develop a specific cessation plan.
5. Provide a list of programs (detailed by phone number, address, method, and cost) and have available handouts (for instance the National Cancer Institute's or American Lung Association's self-help smoking cessation materials).
6. Follow up and provide encouragement and support.
7. Prepare for relapse.

For participants who simply refuse to quit at this time, ask them if you can ask about quitting in the future, and do so. Individuals not willing to quit at one time may change their mind later on and will benefit from a kind but firm continued reminder of the importance of stopping.

DIET

The chief goals of dietary change are often to:

1. reduce or maintain body weight,
2. reduce elevated plasma LDL-cholesterol or VLDL-cholesterol, and
3. reduce blood pressure.

These goals are brought about through appropriate changes in calories, saturated fat, cholesterol, and salt intake as suggested by the Senate Select Committee's Dietary Goals for the Nation. A person's excess calorie, sodium, or cholesterol intake develops over a long time. Permanent adoption of an eating style that helps a person lose weight, lower cholesterol, and/or reduce sodium intake, usually requires a slow but persistent change in eating habits. The following steps may be useful.

1. Provide information to the participant as to the need for change and the advantages of doing so.
2. Establish a baseline of the participant's current dietary intake. Computerized 24-hour dietary intake programs, food diaries, or a 4–7 day recall can be used for this purpose.
3. Establish concrete short-term goals and make committments to achieving these goals.
4. Provide appropriate nutrition, food preparation, and other relevant material.
5. Continue to follow the participant's progress in reaching the short-term goals. As short-term goals are reached, new goals should be established until the long-term dietary changes are reached.

A well-trained exercise leader may be able to provide assistance for achieving the above steps; consultation with a dietician is also important.

BODY COMPOSITION

Available evidence indicates that the prevalence of moderate or severe obesity is high. Although the best measure of obesity is percent body fat, most studies have focused on total body weight. On the basis of weight, one survey indicates that approximately 5% of men and 7% of women are severely obese. While a few people are overweight because of hormonal or other physical disorders, the majority who are excessively fat exercise too little relative to caloric intake. Permanent weight loss can occur by decreasing food consumption and by increasing energy expended through physical activity. Many studies have shown that the adoption of a physical activity program is the best predictor of long-term weight loss and its subsequent maintenance. Many self-help, therapist-aided, or group programs which teach new eating habits and encourage physical activity are available, and lead to a realistic and safe rate of weight loss of approximately 1 kg a week.

A participant can be helped with a weight loss program in several ways.

1. Emphasize the importance of gradual weight loss based on changes in the diet (decreased caloric intake) and increased physical activity.

2. Review the participant's past successes and failures with weight loss.
3. Establish realistic short and long-term goals. Avoid fad diets or fasts.
4. Provide appropriate written support and instructional materials.
5. Prepare the client for relapses (for instance, not to become discouraged with a high calorie binge) or plateaus of weight loss (more exercise, or fewer calories might be indicated).
6. Continue to monitor the person's progress and provide support and encouragement.

Since change in body composition should be a gradual process, with occasional lack of progress likely to occur, the exercise leader should assume a patient, nonjudgmental attitude. See Chapters 3 and 5 for additional guidelines for a proper weight loss program.

STRESS MANAGEMENT

Stress management techniques aimed at altering physiologic variables (like blood pressure or heart rate), inducing a general state of relaxation and well-being, changing behavior patterns, enhancing coping mechanisms, or combinations of these techniques are becoming increasingly popular. Stress management programs include avoidance techniques where the participant avoids the stressful situation, adjustment/adaptation techniques where the participant copes more appropriately with the stressor, or alteration techniques like relaxation and biofeedback which normalizes physiology. The specific stress management techniques to be used remain controversial. Most people can easily learn a relaxation procedure; other stress management techniques may require more intensive instruction and practice.

REFERENCES

Blumenthal JA, Califf R, Williams RS, Hindman M: Cardiac rehabilitation: A new frontier for behavioral medicine. *Cardiac Rehab, 3*:637–656, 1983.

Enelow AJ, Swisher SN: *Interviewing and Patient Care.* New York: Oxford, 1979.

Jenkins D: An approach to the diagnosis and treatment of problems of health related behavior. *Int Health Educ, 22* (suppl): 1–24, 1979.

Martin JE, Dubbert PM: Exercise applications and promotion in behavioral medicine: Current status and future directions. *J Consult Clin Psych, 50*:1004–1017, 1982.

Melamed BG, Siegel LJ: *Behavioral Medicine: Practical Applications in Health Care.* New York: Springer, 1980.

7

Program Administration

Exercise programs and exercise testing laboratories should be organized in accordance with accepted administrative procedures. The material in this chapter pertains primarily to administration of medically oriented programs for higher risk participants. Many of the recommendations in this chapter are also applicable to preventive exercise programs offered in the university or worksite settings. It is recommended that medically supervised exercise programs adhere to the following administrative guidelines.

MANAGEMENT STRUCTURE AND FUNCTION

Effective program administration is enhanced through well-defined organizational relationships which clearly identify specific personnel responsibilities and sources of authority. Ultimate accountability for the program should rest with a governing body-advisory committee composed of appropriate professionals who contribute their collective knowledge toward development and operation of the program. This governing body should include individuals whose expertise will add to the success of the program. Such persons may include health educators, dieticians, attorneys, insurance experts, business and accounting advisors, and local health agency representatives to name a few. The policies and procedures adopted by this body provide the guidelines for the development and operation of the exercise program and the delegation of responsibilities to appropriate administrators. Program guidelines should be reviewed and updated on an annual basis in order to integrate new techniques and delete those segments of the program which appear to be ineffective. "Five-year program goals and objectives" should be written in order to prepare for future growth and program changes.

The position of program director requires training and experience in leadership, planning, delegation of authority, and assumption of responsibility. The effective administrator has a broad academic understanding, insight into human relationships, practical intelligence, and a strong commitment to exercise program goals.

FINANCIAL CONCERNS

Income and expenditure accounting procedures are established within guidelines determined by the program governing board. A board member with accounting capabilities will facilitate a development of practical policies. Some financial planning is assured by a realistic and accurate appraisal of conditions affecting the program. Budget development should follow a reasonable sequence which includes inventory, staff input, analysis and review, submission and approval, revision, direct and indirect expense revenue projection and budget administration. Regular income sources must be managed carefully to ensure a consistent cash flow in balance with projected expenses.

The major source of income for preventive and rehabilitative exercise programs is through participant fees. These exercise programs should use materials which explain the program fees to the participant, referring physician and/or the insurance carriers prior to enrollment. Medicare, Medicaid and Vocational Rehabilitation agencies should be considered as alternative income sources, developed and utilized. Such income may be reserved for research, capital expenditures and contingencies. Line item accountability is the most accurate method of bookkeeping and with standard record-keeping practices provides reliable data for future financial planning.

LEGAL CONSIDERATIONS

It is essential that standing orders from a physician and approved procedures be developed through careful study of national and local practices and with the guidance of medical and legal advisors to provide the best standards of reasonable and prudent care. Constant monitoring of personnel, activity selection, and/or environmental conditions along with regular inservice training of staff should be provided within these standards. Specific policies for protection of the rights, confidentiality and safety of patients must be developed and understood by all staff persons. Such policies include, but are not limited to, the obtaining of informed consent (see Appendices A and C) (the basis of which provides documentation of the voluntary assumption of risk by the participant) and developing standing orders for emergency procedures. All such policies should be presented to program participants in written form prior to their participation. Guidelines for safe exercise, exercise prescription, early warning signs of an impending heart attack, facility rules and regulations are a few items which can be covered in a participant handbook.

Administrators must be aware that state statutes which govern the practice of medicine are generally restrictive, vary widely in scope and, if violated, can result in lawsuits. Self-protective procedures, (1) in-service training to be informed of current accepted procedures, (2) employing certified or licensed staff persons, (all medical supervisory staff should be certified in Advanced Cardiac Life Support or the equivalent) and non-medical supervisory staff should be certified in Basic Life Support as designated by the American Heart Association or the equivalent, (3) periodic recertification of personnel and (4) securing satisfactory limits of liability insurance are also important. Written documentation of problems and staff recommendations are a necessary part of good medical management and legal coverage. All such documentations should be filed and kept per state requirement.

Careful screening and monitoring of participants and the utilization of written documentation of procedures provides for a safe and "legal" program.

FACILITY AND EQUIPMENT REQUIREMENTS

Careful matching of program activities, facilities, and equipment will contribute to the continued success of an exercise program. Facility recommendations include:

1. a walking-running area with safe traffic patterns,
2. a testing area which is quiet, electrically grounded, and offers easy access for emergency situations,
3. an educational area where lectures, demonstrations, films and study materials can be made available,
4. a private counseling area,

5. an administrative area where records and other office materials are secure,
6. emergency equipment including a defibrillator, and
7. locker rooms and restrooms which are well-ventilated, easily accessible, secure and supervised.

Specific equipment and supply requirements are determined by the type of program offered. The administrator should maintain records of suppliers, warranty agreements, operating manuals, replacement availabilities and costs. A complete preventive maintenance program that includes calibration checks is recommended for optimal equipment performance. Local fire codes and regulations should be posted along with emergency checks, exercise equipment repair, fire drills and emergency evacuation practice should be kept. All staff personnel should be held responsible for educating participants and enforcing the safe use of facilities and equipment in accordance with procedures approved by the governing body.

PUBLIC RELATIONS

The function of public relations is to influence opinion through communications to participants and within the community. Public relations includes publicity, advertising and promotion. It is essentially an administrative responsibility to evaluate attitudes and to identify interest in, and promote community understanding of the exercise program. Information disseminated must be timely, accurate and comprehensible if it is to positively reflect the program. Carefully planned public relations will enable the administrator to identify community resources and obstacles. These data are essential for coordinating program efforts and interagency cooperation. Community service organizations can provide the speaking engagements and informal contacts for distributing program information which might lead to potential sources of funding. Newsletter, radio, television, workshops, seminars, news releases, health fairs, and demonstration projects are excellent media for presenting ideas, securing new participants and describing current events. Identification of sources of referral can help to guide your efforts in promotion. Maximizing efforts in those areas which appear most likely to result in new program participation will be a tremendous time-saver and more productive. Probably the most influential source of public relations is through word-of-mouth. Though this source is not directly controllable, it is best developed through high quality program administration and through the professionalism displayed during program operations.

PROGRAM EVALUATION

Program evaluation is an ongoing administrative function that should be developed from several sources. Initially, the administrator should evaluate program effectiveness in terms of cost, staff productivity, public image and, most importantly, service to the participants and community. This evaluation is usually influenced by objective and subjective input from the program governing body. Second, the participants should be required to provide an evaluation of program effectiveness. This can be easily accomplished by a simple questionnaire mailed annually to all current and past participants.

Assessment of participants' attitude, knowledge and behavior change are useful supplement to the usual physiologic measurements included in most programs. Measureable goals for overall behavior change are particularly useful. An example is setting a goal of a given percentage of smokers in the program expected to maintain cessation of 6 months, or a given percentage of adherence or attendance of exercise sessions.

QUALITY CONTROL CHECKLIST

The following checklist gives the parameters which have been developed by the American College of Sports Medicine as guidelines for exercise testing laboratories and cardiac rehabilitation programs. The program director might use these parameters to develop a quality control checklist for internal use. This list is not intended to be an instrument for external evaluation, but merely to provide guidelines for the program.

CHECKLIST FOR QUALITY CONTROL OF EXERCISE TESTING LABORATORIES AND CARDIAC REHABILITATION PROGRAMS

Organizational Structure and Mechanics

Organizational chart, business practices, billing procedures, office records, patient files, primary physician contact, recruitment of patients, recruitment of staff, forms.

Patient Procedures

Referral process, qualifications, histories, exclusions/contraindications, orientation, entrance procedures, exit policy.

Assessment Procedures

Exercise test, informed consent, exercise test protocols, exercise test termination criteria, ancillary tests, equipment meeting AHA standards (treadmill, bicycle ergometer, ECG), personnel (ACSM certification of MD, RN, PT, physiologist, technologist, exercise specialist), ECG interpreted by physician, adequate exercise test interpretation (HR, BP, symptom responses) work capacity identified and recorded and ST-T changes, dysrrhythmias recorded.

Equipment

Motor-driven treadmill, calibrated bicycle ergometer, and/or step ergometer with height stop (meeting AHA standards), ECG machine (meeting AHA standards) oscilloscope visible at working distance, blood pressure cuff, stethoscope, medical kit or crash cart stocked with drugs which are updated, defibrillator present and tested before each day of use.

In-Hospital Rehabilitation Program (Phase I)

Initial evaluation, entrance/rejection criteria, exercise prescription methods, facilities, equipment, personnel, organization of sessions, exercise variety, exercise progressions, monitoring exercise, data recording/reporting to MD, modification of exercise, patient files, non-exercise aspects (nutrition/diet program, vocational counseling, psychologic counseling, occupational therapy, patient/family education), exit criteria.

Outpatient Program (Phase II or III)

The same as Phase I with home exercise program, patient followup, ability to monitor HR, BP, ECG, and symptoms, use training heart rate as index of training, have documented criteria for indications, contraindications, precautions, separate protocols for uncomplicated and complicated subsets, have primary exercise modes, assessment of progress, record keeping and reporting, exit criteria.

Emergency Procedures

Qualifications of personnel (current CPR certification), assignment of personnel during emergency/written procedures, emergency equipment and supplies, supply update, equipment testing, in-service updating, incident recording/reporting procedures, locker room coverage, paramedic notification, adequacy of paramedic response time, awareness of closest emergency room for advanced life support, ability to contact family or referring physician on site.

Qualifications and Responsibilities of Personnel

Credentials on file, peer review, in-service sessions/staff meetings, CME update, minimal job qualifications.

Year-end Summaries

Total number of exercise tests, exercise sessions, ECGs, cardiovascular incidents (acute MIs, cardiac arrests, dysrrhythmias, and events requiring contact with the patient's physician), and other services.

Organizational Structure

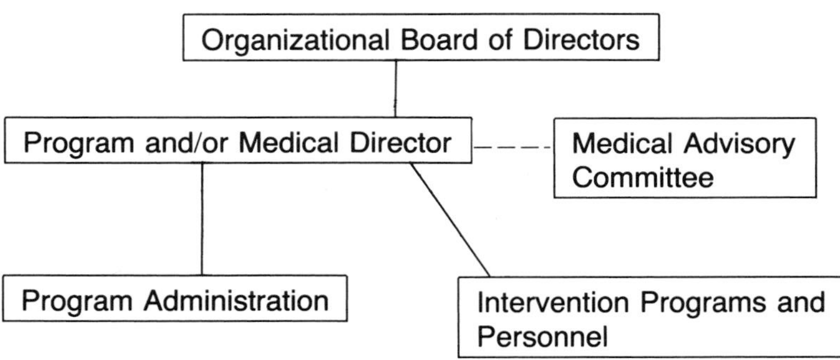

An organizational structure such as the one shown above provides for a clear delineation of financial/administrative versus medical management and intervention responsibilities. This is an important concept as most programs have definite medical as well as administrative needs and concerns.

A strong link between the Medical and/or Program Director and Program Administrator is necessary because of the important input they both have relative to continuing management and future growth. Many other organizational patterns are possible. What is important is that there are clear lines of accountability, there is overall medical direction, and areas of responsibility are clearly delineated.

SUGGESTED READING

Exercise Standards Book, Dallas: American Heart Association, 1979.

8

The Role of Physicians in Exercise Programs

Physicians have an important role in exercise testing, especially in high risk or symptomatic populations. Physicians involved in exercise testing need not be cardiologists or internists, but they must have diagnostic skills that include recognition of the history, physical and laboratory test conditions where exercise testing must be modified or is contraindicated. These conditions are outlined elsewhere in these guidelines. Physicians must also be especially aware of effects of cardiorespiratory drugs on the ECG and on heart rate and blood pressure responses to exercise performance and training. The physician should be comfortable in recognizing specific ECG abnormalities that may be encountered in exercise testing. These include such abnormalities as atrial and ventricular dysrhythmias, ST segment depression and elevation, left and right bundle branch block, and heart block.

Physicians should recognize the value of a maximal exercise test in measurement of fitness, provision of information for the exercise prescription, motivation of patients to exercise, and in diagnostic assessment for determining the likelihood of the presence of coronary disease. An exercise tolerance test can be an invaluable extension of a physical examination to detect latent disease and assessing a patient's functional capacity. Physicians should be familiar with the various exercise protocols and how to select the appropriate protocol for the individual patient.

The ability to communicate with patients is an essential skill for physicians involved in exercise testing. Physicians hold a unique position for teaching and motivating patients about exercise and its benefits, and this advantage should not be lost because of busy schedules or less than desirable communication skills.

Physician involvement in all aspects of preventive and rehabilitative exercise programs is to be encouraged. Ideally, physicians would be involved from the earliest stages of program development. If local physicians only have the skills and interest required for a supporting role, a program may be initiated by an exercise program director, exercise specialist, and where appropriate by a health fitness instructor or director. Under these circumstances, physician guidance of the exercise program may be obtained from the development of a medical advisory committee, a component of the governing body recommended for program administration.

It is beneficial in any exercise program for the physician to take a leadership role. The physician is responsible for policies regulating the safety and well-being of participants by insuring that emergency management programs are in place and staff training occurs regularly. The physician will also function in the role of diagnostician, decision maker, teacher, and counselor as well as assist in public relations. It is essential that physicians recognize the professional skills and competencies of exercise program directors, exercise specialist, exercise test technologists and health fitness instructors/directors and delegate appropriate responsibilities.

Private physicians who are not involved in group exercise programs have extensive opportunities for exercise testing and training in individual patients. They are in a unique position to motivate their patients to begin and continue exercise programs. When private physicians give their patients exercise recommendations, they should be careful to give specific advice on types of exercise, frequency, intensity, and duration, rather than simply telling patients to get more exercise. Physicians without interest or expertise in exercise testing and training should seek competent referral networks in their communities in order to give their patients the benefit of qualified testing and exercise training.

Physicians involved with occupational medicine often have opportunities to encourage and direct corporate fitness programs. These individuals may be instrumental in obtaining funding and management support for such programs as well as in planning and directing the programs themselves.

Many physicians have been certified as preventive and rehabilitative program directors and as exercise specialists, but certification is not considered a necessary prerequisite for those who wish to assume medical direction of programs. The certification programs of the American College of Sports Medicine can evaluate the expertise and competence of a physician as a program director of a preventive or rehabilitative exercise program, but competence as a medical specialist is evaluated by the American Board of Medical Specialities and similar certifying organizations in other countries.

Physicians involved in exercise programs must be licensed to practice and should be protected by professional liability insurance. They should maintain certification in advanced cardiac life support techniques or an equivalent (as the team emergency and safety leader).

9

Certification of Preventive and Rehabilitation Exercise Program Personnel

There are certain functions which include specific knowledges, skills and competencies for each of the five categories of certification: (1) exercise test technologist, (2) health fitness instructor, (3) exercise specialist, (4) health fitness director, and (5) exercise program director. There are progressive levels of knowledges, skills, and competencies required within each of the categories of certification. The exercise test technologist must demonstrate competence in exercise testing of various individuals in states of illness and health; the health fitness instructor must demonstrate competence in exercise testing, designing and executing an exercise program, leading exercise and organizing and operating fitness facilities for healthy individuals or those with controlled diseases; the exercise specialist, in addition to the competencies expected of the exercise test technologist and health fitness instructor, must demonstrate competency in implementing exercise prescriptions and leading exercise for individuals with known cardiovascular, pulmonary or metabolic disease; the health fitness director in addition to the competencies expected of a health fitness instructor must demonstrate competence in preventive program administration, supervising staff, and program evaluation. The exercise program director, in addition to the competencies expected of the exercise test technologist, health fitness instructor, exercise specialist and health fitness director must demonstrate competence in administering preventive and rehabilitative programs, designing and implementing exercise programs, educating staff and community, and designing and conducting research.

Minimal competencies have been outlined according to behavioral objectives. A behavioral objective is a statement indicating what a person should be able to do following some unit of instruction or study. Two types of objectives are presented here. The General Objective (GO) describes the unobservable mental process, while the Specific Learning Objective (SLO) describes the behavior in observable terms.

PREVENTIVE AND REHABILITATIVE EXERCISE TEST TECHNOLOGIST

The primary responsibility of the exercise test technologist is to administer exercise tests safely in order to obtain reliable and valid data. The exercise test technologist should demonstrate appropriate knowledge of functional anatomy, exercise physiology, pathophysiology, electrocardiography, and psychology in order to perform tasks such as preparing the exercise test station for administration of exercise tests, preliminary screening of the participant for the exercise test, administering tests and recording data, implementing emergency procedures when necessary, summarizing test data, and communicating the test results to the exercise specialists, program directors and physicians. After a participant's medical evaluation is received from a referring physician, the exercise test technologist may administer an exercise test independently or based on the health status and age of the participant (Chapter 2). The technologist must be able to recognize contraindications to exercise testing found in preliminary screening, recognize abnormal responses during the exercise test and during recovery, and respond appropriately.

While there is no prerequisite experience or level of education required for the exercise test technologist, study in the fields of the biological sciences, physical education and health related professions are examples of appropriate training for those desiring certification. Although not mandatory, work experience under a physician or exercise program director would be a valuable asset to the certification applicant. The certified exercise test technologist, working with individual participants during exercise and assisting in other roles in preventive and rehabilitative exercise programs, may gain the necessary experience to apply for the exercise specialist certification.

BEHAVIORAL OBJECTIVES

The exercise test technologist will demonstrate competency in exercise testing. This includes the following general and specific learning outcomes:

HEALTH APPRAISAL AND TESTING TECHNIQUES

GO

The exercise test technologist will demonstrate skills and have knowledge in administering an exercise test; including but not limited to equipment calibration, patient screening and patient instruction, an understanding of the components of the physical examination, selecting a test protocol, recording test data, and case summary.

SLO

Describe the techniques used to calibrate a(n) motor driven treadmill, cycle ergometer, arm ergometer, electrocardiographic recorder, and mercury or anaeroid sphygmomanometer.

SLO

Perform a routine screening procedure prior to testing. Procedures include history taking (particularly facts relevant to exercise test); obtaining informed consent; explaining procedures and protocol for the exercise test; recognizing the contraindications to an exercise test; and providing results of screening procedures to the physician and indicate participants for whom physician supervision is required.

SLO

Describe the components of a physical exam and their significance to exercise testing.

SLO

Perform routine tasks prior to exercise testing, including:

A. Taking a standard 12 lead electrocardiogram on a participant in a supine posture, in an upright posture, and during hyperventilation;
B. Accurately recording right and left arm and arterial blood pressure in different body postures.
C. Demonstrate the ability to instruct the test participant in the use of a rating of perceived exertion (RPE) scale during the exercise test.

SLO

Perform an exercise test.

A. Structure an exercise test protocol (continuous or discontinuous) with reference to the initial exercise intensity in METs, and increments of exercise intensity in METs for the cycle ergometer, arm ergometer and treadmill according to the participant's age, sex, weight, estimated level of fitness, and health status including modifications for pulmonary patients.
B. Record appropriate measurements and participant responses, e.g., symptoms, ECG, blood pressure, heart rate, and perceived exertion at appropriate intervals during the test.
C. Identify possible test endpoints (e.g. signs and symptoms, or

inappropriate responses, workload, HR or perceived exertion) which would terminate the exercise test for healthy or high-risk individuals, or for coronary bypass or myocardial infarction patients undergoing either pre or post-discharge testing.

SLO
Demonstrate an ability to measure resting pulmonary parameters, e.g. FEV_1, FVC and respiratory frequency.

SLO
Describe standard scales used to evaluate dyspnea and functional class of the pulmonary patient.

SLO
Calculate and organize test data in a seqential manner.

A. Transform or reduce data preparing it for use by the physician, program director, or exercise specialist.

GO
The exercise test technologist will demonstrate knowledge in the operation and administration of an exercise testing facility.

SLO
Describe a plan for organizing an exercise testing laboratory and include facilities and equipment.

SLO
Describe a plan outlining the events of a typical testing day's activities.

EMERGENCY PROCEDURES

GO
The exercise test technologist will demonstrate competency in responding, with appropriate emergency procedures, to situations which might arise prior to, during, and after administration of exercise tests.

SLO
Present valid CPR certification credentials.

SLO
List and describe the use of emergency equipment which should be present in an exercise testing laboratory.

SLO
Identify and describe the use of emergency drugs which should be available during exercise testing.

SLO
Demonstrate ability to assist a physician during an emergency situation.

SLO
Demonstrate competency in verifying operating status of and maintaining emergency equipment.

SLO Describe emergency procedures for a preventive and rehabilitative exercise testing program.

FUNCTIONAL ANATOMY

GO

The exercise test technologist will demonstrate a knowledge of functional anatomy.

SLO

Identify anatomic sites for selected measures associated with the exercise test.

A. Locate the appropriate sites for the limb and chest leads of the ECG.
B. Locate the brachial artery and position the cuff for the measurement of blood pressure.
C. Locate anatomic landmarks that might be required in determining the peripheral pulses.
D. Locate anatomic landmarks that might be required in anthropometry.
E. Locate the anatomic landmarks used during cardiopulmonary resuscitation and emergency procedures.

SLO

Identify the major features of cardiopulmonary anatomy, specifically, chambers, valves, vessels, conduction, tracheobronchial tree.

EXERCISE PHYSIOLOGY

GO

The exercise test technologist will demonstrate a knowledge of exercise physiology.

SLO

Define aerobic and anaerobic metabolism.

SLO

Describe the cardiorespiratory responses to postural changes and exercise including heart rate (HR), stroke volume (SV), cardiac output (Q), blood pressure (SBP, DBP) and ventilatory response.

A. Contrast the cardiorespiratory responses to postural changes before and after exercise testing.

SLO

List modifications to exercise testing.

A. List physiologic considerations in the selection of different modes of ergometry, i.e., treadmill, cycle, or arm ergometer.
B. Describe the principle of specificity as it relates to the mode of testing.
C. List the advantages and disadvantages of continuous vs. discontinuous tests.
D. Describe the physiologic importance of the warm-up, rate of exercise progression, and the implications of various post-exercise procedures as these relate to exercise testing.
E. List the effects of temperature and humidity upon the physiologic response to exercise testing.
F. List the signs and symptoms that are used in designating the endpoint of an exercise test.

PATHOPHYSIOLOGY

GO
The exercise test technologist will demonstrate a knowledge of the basic pathophysiology of ischemic heart diseases.

SLO
Define ischemia and explain the methods that are used to record and measure ischemic responses. List the effects of ischemic heart diseases (including myocardial infarction) upon performance and safety during an exercise test.

SLO
Define hypotension and hypertension.

SLO
List major risk factors for ischemic heart diseases.

SLO
Explain why blood pressure should be monitored during the exercise test.

SLO
Discuss the factors that effect myocardial oxygen supply and demand and describe the effects of atherosclerosis, coronary arterial spasm and acute exercise on each of these factors.

SLO
List special considerations necessary when testing participants with obesity, diabetes, renal disease, pulmonary disease, asthma, orthopedic, neurologic problems, hypertension or stroke.

SLO
Describe the effects of the following classifications of drugs on the ECG, heart rate and blood pressure. (See Appendix B).

A. Antianginal (nitrates, beta blockers, etc.)
B. Antiarrhythmic
C. Anticoagulant
D. Antiplatelet aggregation
E. Lipid lowering drugs
F. Antihypertensive (diuretics, vasodilators, etc.)
G. Digitalis glycosides
H. Calcium channel blocking agents
I. Bronchodilators
J. Tranquilizers, antidepressants, and antianxiety drugs

SLO
Define emphysema, asthma, chronic obstructive pulmonary disease, pulmonary vascular disease, and psychogenic hyperventilation.

ELECTROCARDIOGRAPHY

GO
The exercise test technologist will demonstrate a knowledge of normal and abnormal resting electrocardiograms and be able to recognize

selected ECG abnormalities during the administration of an exercise test.

SLO
Describe the normal resting electrocardiogram.

A. Draw a normal ECG complex and label important waves, intervals, and points.
B. List functional phenomena or events associated with the various segments of the electrocardiogram.

SLO
Identify the ECG changes that are associated with an ischemic response at rest and during exercise.

A. Draw and label ECG complexes that are representative of either subendocardial or transmural ischemia (also called the injury pattern).
B. Define the limits or considerations in terminating an exercise test on the basis of the signs and symptoms of an ischemic response (e.g. ECG changes, cyanosis, angina).

SLO
Identify the ECG changes that are associated with the following abnormalities: arrhythmias; conduction defects; myocardial infarctions.

A. Draw and label ECG complexes that are representative of the following abnormalities:
   1. Acute myocardial infarction.
   2. Resolved (old) myocardial infarction.
   3. Cardiac standstill (ventricular asystole)
   4. Sinus bradycardia (< 60/min.)
   5. Differences between supraventricular and ventricular rhythms.
   6. Premature ventricular complexes (frequency, multifocal, couplets, salvos, and R on T).
   7. Ventricular tachycardia.
   8. Ventricular fibrillation.
   9. Atrioventricular blocks of all degrees.
   10. Atrial fibrillation.
   11. Atrial flutter.
B. Define the limits or considerations in terminating an exercise test on the basis of the ECG abnormalities listed.

SLO
Identify ECG changes that may occur in hyperventilation.

SLO
Identify resting ECG changes associated with diseases other than CHD, such as, hypertensive heart disease, cardiac chamber enlargement, metabolic disorders, pericarditis and pulmonary disease.

HUMAN BEHAVIOR/PSYCHOLOGY

GO
The exercise test technologist will demonstrate knowledge of psychologic factors which may affect exercise participants.

SLO
List six factors which increase anxiety in the exercise testing laboratory and describe how anxiety may be reduced in a participant.

SLO
List potential manifestations of test anxiety which can influence responses to an exercise test.

HUMAN DEVELOPMENT/AGING

GO
The exercise test technologist will demonstrate competence in selecting appropriate test protocol according to the age of the participant.

SLO
Describe adjustments which might be necessary for testing the younger participant, specifically, instructions for the patient and modification of the testing protocol and equipment.

THE PREVENTIVE TRACT: HEALTH/FITNESS PERSONNEL

There are two major categories of certification which have been developed for personnel working in preventive and rehabilitative programs: the *Preventive* and the *Rehabilitative Tracts.* The *Preventive Tract* is designed primarily for those who provide leadership in programs of a preventive nature, for healthy individuals or those with controlled disease. The *Rehabilitative Tract* is designed for professionals who are primarily responsible for working with diseased individuals enrolled in rehabilitative programs. These rehabilitation specialists are also authorized to provide similar leadership in programs of a preventive nature.

Within the *Preventive Tract,* three levels of certification are offered:

Health Fitness Director

Health Fitness Instructor

Fitness Leader/Specialty

Each of the preventive certification levels requires that individuals certified at a given level are responsible for the behavioral objectives of the level(s) below theirs. In addition, a *core* of behavioral objectives has been developed to serve as the foundation for all of the above certification levels. This core contains the desired breadth and depth of knowledges considered to be essential for all preventive personnel.

FITNESS LEADER/SPECIALTY

The individuals certified at this level are considered to be "entry level" personnel who will serve under the leadership of a Health Fitness Instructor and/or a Health Fitness Director. In addition to their command of the core behavioral objectives, these individuals have unique knowledge and skills in a specific area of specialization such as dance exercise, military, law enforcement or other future tracts. The Fitness Leader has primary responsibility in the fitness program as an exercise leader. There are no special educational prerequisites for this level.

HEALTH FITNESS INSTRUCTOR

Certification at the level of Health Fitness Instructor requires a greater depth and breadth of knowledge in each of the areas encompassed by a multidisciplinary approach to prevention. The Health Fitness Instructor has the responsibility of training and/or supervising Fitness Leaders during an exercise program but may also serve as an exercise leader. In addition, the Health Fitness Instructor can serve as a health counselor to participants in need of multiple intervention strategies for lifestyle change. The minimum educational prerequisite is a baccalaureate degree in an allied health field or the equivalent. Candidates for this certification are also expected to have appropriate experience in exercise programming and leadership.

HEALTH FITNESS DIRECTOR

The individual certified at this highest preventive level is required to have a command of the behavioral objectives of the two previous levels and will incorporate the administrative knowledges and skills as the director of a preventive program. The Health Fitness Director should have considerable background and experience with the administrative aspects of preventive programs and also should have leadership qualities which ensure competence in the training and supervision of personnel. The minimum educational prerequisite is a postgraduate degree in an allied health field or the equivalent. In addition, in order to qualify as a Health Fitness Director, an internship or period of practical experience of at least 1 year is required as described in the behavioral objectives.

ACSM PREVENTIVE TRACT: CORE BEHAVIORAL OBJECTIVES

EXERCISE PHYSIOLOGY

GO
The candidate will demonstrate a knowledge of basic exercise physiology.

SLO
Define aerobic and anaerobic metabolism in terms of energy expenditure.

SLO
Describe the role of carbohydrates, fats, and protein as fuels for anaerobic and aerobic performance.

SLO
Describe the normal cardiorespiratory responses to an exercise bout in terms of heart rate, blood pressure, and oxygen consumption. Describe how these responses change with adaptation to chronic exercise training and how men and women may differ in response.

SLO
Define and explain the relationship of METs and Kilocalories to physical activity.

SLO
Describe the heart rate and blood pressure responses to static (isometric), dynamic (isotonic) and isokinetic exercise.

SLO
Define and explain the concept of specificity of exercise conditioning.

SLO
Describe how heart rate is determined by pulse palpation. List precautions in the application of these techniques.

SLO
Calculate predicted maximal heart rate for various ages.

SLO
Define the following terms: ischemia, angina pectoris, premature ventricular contraction, premature atrial contraction, tachycardia, bradycardia, myocardial infarction, Valsalva maneuver, hyperventilation, oxygen consumption, cardiac output, stroke volume, lactic acid, hypertension, high density lipoprotein cholesterol (HDL-C), total cholesterol/high density lipoprotein cholesterol ratio, anemia, bulimia, anorexia nervosa.

SLO
Describe blood pressure responses associated with changes in different body positions.

SLO
Describe the purpose and function of an electrocardiogram.

SLO
Identify the physiologic principles related to warm-up and cool-down.

GO
The candidate will demonstrate an understanding of the basic principles involved in muscular strength, endurance, and flexibility training.

SLO
Identify the physiologic principles related to muscular endurance and strength training: define overload, specificity, use-disuse, progressive resistance.

SLO
Define muscular atrophy, hypertrophy, hyperplasia, concentric and eccentric contractions, sets and repetition.

SLO
Describe the common theories of muscle fatigue and delayed muscle soreness.

SLO
Describe the muscle stretch reflex.

NUTRITION AND WEIGHT MANAGEMENT

GO
The candidate will demonstrate an understanding of basic nutrition and weight management.

SLO
Give the recommended ranges for percent body fat (male and female).

SLO
Contrast the effectiveness of diet plus exercise, diet alone or exercise alone for fat loss or body composition changes.

SLO
Define the following terms: obesity, overweight, underweight, percent fat, lean body mass.

SLO
Describe the procedures for maintaining normal hydration at times of heavy sweating; contrast plain water replacement with the use of special electrolyte drinks.

SLO
Explain the concept of energy balance as it relates to weight control.

SLO

Explain the difference between fat and water soluble vitamins and the potential risk of toxicity with over-supplementation.

SLO

Discuss the inappropriate use of salt tablets, diet pills, protein powders, liquid protein diets and nutritional supplements.

SLO

Discuss the misconceptions of spot reduction and rapid weight loss.

SLO

Be familiar with the Dietary Goals recommended by the Senate Select Committee on Nutrition and Human Needs and the exchange lists of the American Dietetic Association.

SLO

Identify the basic four food groups and give examples of each.

SLO

Describe the interaction of diet and/or exercise as they relate to the blood lipid profile.

EXERCISE PROGRAMMING

GO

The candidate will understand the role of exercise for persons with stable disease or no disease and demonstrate competence in designing and implementing individualized and group exercise programs.

SLO

Given a case study containing the following information: health history, risk factors, medical information, and results of a fitness evaluation, the candidate will be able to:

A. Use these data for recommending appropriate exercise based on proper intensity (training heart rate), duration, frequency, progression, type of physical activity and whether exercise is to be performed in a supervised or unsupervised program.
B. Modify an exercise program (i.e., intensity, duration, etc.) under such environmental conditions as cold, heat, humidity, and altitude.
C. Describe the importance of flexibility and recommend proper exercises for improving range of motion of all major joints. Describe the difference between static and dynamic (ballistic) stretching.
D. Describe and demonstrate appropriate exercise used in warm-up and cool-down.
E. Describe and demonstrate exercises for the improvement of muscular strength and endurance.
F. Describe the difference between interval and continuous training.
G. Describe the relationship of the heart rate response to physical activity and perceived exertion. Demonstrate various methods for monitoring physical effort such as heart rate, blood pressure, and perceived exertion.

H. Describe the signs and symptoms of over-exercising which would indicate the need to decrease the intensity, duration, or frequency of an exercise session.

SLO

Explain the effects of the following categories of substances on exercise responses: beta blockers, nitroglycerin, diuretics, antihypertensives, antihistamines, tranquilizers, alcohol, diet pills, cold tablets, illicit drugs and caffeine.

SLO

Explain appropriate modifications in exercise programs due to acute illness, (colds, etc.), and controlled conditions (such as diabetes, chronic obstructive pulmonary diseases, allergies, hypertension, and cardiovascular disease) that a physician might recommend for your exercising client.

EMERGENCY PROCEDURES

GO

The candidate will demonstrate competence in basic life support and implementation of first aid procedures which may be necessary during or after exercise.

SLO

Possess current cardiopulmonary (CPR) certification or equivalent credentials.

SLO

Demonstrate an understanding of appropriate emergency procedures (i.e., telephone procedures, preconceived written emergency plan, personnel responsibilities, etc.).

SLO

Understand basic first aid procedures for heat cramps, heat exhaustion, heat stroke, lacerations, incisions, puncture wound, abrasion, contusion, simple-compound fractures, bleeding/shock, hypoglycemia/hyperglycemia, sprains/strains, and fainting.

HEALTH APPRAISAL AND FITNESS EVALUATION TECHNIQUES

GO

The candidate will demonstrate or identify appropriate techniques for health appraisal and use of fitness evaluations.

SLO

Demonstrate knowledge of health history appraisal to obtain information on past and present medical history, prescribed medication, activity patterns, nutritional habits, stress and anxiety levels, family history of heart disease, smoking history, and alcohol and illicit drug use.

SLO

Demonstrate the ability to interview individuals on health hazards such as positive family history, chest pain/chest discomfort, orthopedic limitations, present activity levels.

SLO

Demonstrate the ability to measure pulse rate accurately both at rest and during exercise.

SLO

Describe appropriate tests for assessment of cardiovascular fitness.

SLO

Identify the difference between maximal and submaximal cardiovascular evaluations.

SLO

Describe appropriate tests for assessment of muscular strength, muscular endurance and flexibility assessment.

SLO

Identify appropriate criteria for discontinuing a fitness evaluation.

SLO

Identify techniques used to determine body composition.

SLO

Identify the needs for retest evaluations for participants in exercise programs and the appropriate time intervals for reevaluation.

EXERCISE LEADERSHIP

GO

The candidate will demonstrate an understanding of principles and practices of leading physical activity.

SLO

Explain appropriate modifications in the exercise program due to musculoskeletal problems, e.g., arthritis, overweight, chondromalacia, lower back discomfort.

SLO

Describe the components of an exercise class or session from the time the participant enters, until the end of the class.

GO

The candidate will be competent in exercise leadership.

SLO

Describe appropriate exercise apparel for a variety of activities and environmental conditions.

SLO

Describe methods to establish appropriate exercise intensity.

SLO

Identify inappropriate exercise responses which would indicate termination of the exercise session.

SLO

Describe the myths and dangers pertaining to body composition changes and/or improved fitness in relation to the following: saunas, vibrating belts, body wraps, electric muscle stimulators (legal implications), and sweat suits.

SLO

Describe the dangers and precautions of the following exercises: straight leg sit ups, double leg raises, full squats, hurdlers stretch exercise, plough exercise, back hyperextension, and standing straight leg toe touch.

HUMAN BEHAVIOR/PSYCHOLOGY

GO

The candidate will demonstrate an understanding of basic behavioral psychology, group dynamics, and learning techniques.

SLO

Given a series of hypothetical situations involving exercise program participants, the candidate will:

A. Describe the appropriate motivational counseling, behavioral techniques and teaching techniques used in conducting exercise and promoting lifestyle changes.
B. Describe how to manage the group facilitator, comedian, chronic complainer, and disruptor.
C. Define each of the following terms: behavior modification, reinforcement, goal setting, motivation, social support, and peer group pressure.
D. Describe factors affecting the learning process by use of part-whole and progressive learning theories.

SLO

Demonstrate and describe an understanding of counseling skills to motivate an individual to begin an exercise program, enhance exercise adherence, and return to regular exercise.

HUMAN DEVELOPMENT/AGING

GO

The candidate will demonstrate an understanding of the special problems of human development and aging.

SLO

Describe the natural changes that occur from childhood through adolescence and aging in the following: skeletal muscle, bone structure, maximal oxygen uptake, grip strength, flexibility, heart rate, and body composition.

SLO

Identify common orthopedic problems of the adolescent and older participant and explain how an exercise program could be modified to avoid aggravation of these problems.

SLO

Identify the predominant psychologic factors involved in the aging process.

SLO

Describe the physiologic effects of the following factors across the age range: smoking, hypertension, obesity, stress, substance abuse, chronic and acute exercise.

FUNCTIONAL ANATOMY AND KINESIOLOGY

GO
The candidate will demonstrate a knowledge of human functional anatomy and kinesiology.

SLO
Explain the properties and function of bone, muscle and connective tissue.

SLO
Describe the basic anatomy of the heart, cardiovascular system and respiratory system.

SLO
Identify major bones and muscle groups.

SLO
Describe the action of major muscle groups, e.g. trapezius, pectoralis major, latissimus dorsi, biceps, triceps, abdominals, erector spinae, gluteus maximus, quadriceps, hamstrings, gastronemius, tibialis anterior.

GO
The candidate will demonstrate a knowledge of concepts in the prevention, recognition, and management of injury associated with physical activity participation.

SLO
Define the following terms: shin splints, tennis elbow, stress fracture, bursitis and tendonitis, supination, pronation, flexion, extension, adduction, abduction and hyperextension.

SLO
Explain the use of rest, cold, compression and elevation in the initial treating of athletic injuries.

SLO
Discuss the application of heat in the long term treatment of athletic injuries.

SLO
Explain low back syndrome and describe exercises used to prevent this problem.

RISK FACTOR IDENTIFICATION

GO
The candidate will identify risk factors which may require consultation with medical or allied health professionals prior to participation in physical activity or prior to major increases in physical activity intensities and habits.

SLO
Identify primary and secondary risk factors for coronary heart disease which may be favorably modified by regular and appropriate physical activity habits.

SLO
Identify major risk factors which may require further consideration prior to participation in physical activity habits.

SLO
Be familiar with the plasma cholesterol levels for various ages as recommended by the National Institutes of Health Consensus Statement.

SLO
Identify the following cardiovascular risk factors or conditions which may require consultation with medical or allied health professionals prior to participation in physical activity or prior to a major increase in physical activity intensities and habits: inappropriate resting, exercise and recovery HR and BPs; new discomfort or changes in the pattern of discomfort in the chest area, neck, shoulder or arm with exercise or at rest; heart murmurs; myocardial infarction; fainting or dizzy spells; claudication; ischemia.

SLO
Identify the following respiratory risk factors which may require consultation with medical or allied health professionals prior to participation in physical activity or prior to major increases in physical activity intensities and habits: extreme breathlessness after mild exertion or during sleep; asthma; exercise-induced asthma; bronchitis; emphysema.

SLO
Identify the following metabolic risk factors which may require consultation with medical or allied health professionals prior to participation in physical activity or prior to major increases in physical activity intensities and habits: body weight more than 20% above optimal; thyroid disease; diabetes.

SLO
Identify the following musculoskeletal risk factors which may require consultation with medical or allied health professionals prior to physical activity or prior to major increases in physical activity intensities and habits: osteoarthritis, rheumatoid arthritis; low back pain; prosthesis-artificial joints.

HEALTH FITNESS INSTRUCTOR: BEHAVIORAL OBJECTIVES

EXERCISE PHYSIOLOGY

GO
The fitness instructor will demonstrate an understanding of exercise physiology.

SLO
Describe the primary difference between aerobic and anaerobic metabolism and their relative importance in exercise programs.

SLO
Define the properties of cardiac muscle, the generation of the action potential, and normal pathways of conduction.

SLO
Identify and describe the relationship between resting values and the normal response to increasing work intensity, (i.e. heart rate (HR), stroke volume (SV), cardiac output (Q), arteriovenous O_2 difference (a-v O_2 diff), O_2 uptake (VO_2), systolic and diastolic blood pressure (SBP, DBP), minute ventilation (V_E), tidal volume (TV), breathing frequency (f).

SLO
Define and explain the concept of the Metabolic Equivalent Unit (MET) and Kcal. Calculate the energy cost in METs and Kcal for given exercise intensities in stepping exercise, bicycle ergometry, and during horizontal and grade walking and running.

SLO
Identify MET equivalents for various sport, recreational and work tasks.

SLO
Explain the difference in the cardiorespiratory responses to static (isometric) exercise compared with dynamic (isotonic) exercise; include possible hazards of isometric exercise for sedentary or asymptomatic adults.

SLO
Explain the specificity of conditioning and the physiologic differences among cardiorespiratory, endurance, and muscular strength conditioning.

SLO
Describe and demonstrate acceptable laboratory and field exercise test protocols from which functional capacity or Vo_2 max determinations or estimations may be obtained.

SLO
Define the following terms: apnea, dyspnea, hyperemia, respiratory alkalosis and acidosis, hypoxia, orthostatic hypotension, arterial pressures, calorimetry, hyperpnea, hypoventilation.

SLO
Describe the physiologic implications of active and passive warm-up and cool-down.

SLO
Describe the energy continuum with reference to aerobic and anaerobic metabolism during various intensities of work.

SLO
Describe the implications of anaerobic threshold in physical conditioning programs.

SLO

Define and demonstrate reciprocal innervation and its relationship to proprioceptive neuromuscular facilitation (PNF).

SLO

Discuss the physical and psychologic signs of overtraining.

SLO

Define the properties of skeletal muscle.

NUTRITION AND WEIGHT CONTROL

SLO

Identify guidelines for caloric intake for an individual desiring to lose or gain weight.

SLO

Calculate ideal body weight based upon body composition evaluation of lean body weight and fat weight.

EXERCISE PROGRAMMING

SLO

Describe and discuss the advantages/disadvantages and the implementation of interval and continuous conditioning programs.

SLO

Describe the most effective methods for accurate monitoring of exercise heart rate and physical effort and demonstrate specific functional evaluations.

SLO

Describe the precautions taken before exposure to or in preparation for altitude, different ambient temperatures and humidities.

SLO

Describe and demonstrate specific flexibility exercises for inclusion in a warm-up program.

SLO

Describe and design the use and implementation of circuit training program in a health enhancement program.

SLO

Describe special precautions and modifications of exercise programming for special populations (i.e. diabetics, arthritics).

EMERGENCY PROCEDURES

GO

The Health Fitness Instructor will demonstrate competence in the use, maintenance, and updating of appropriate emergency equipment, supplies, and patient transport plans.

SLO

Teach the principles and techniques used in cardiopulmonary resuscitation.

SLO
Demonstrate the emergency procedures, equipment, and materials needed during exercise testing, fitness evaluations, and exercise sessions.

SLO
Discuss the individual responsibility and legal implications related to emergency care.

SLO
Design and update emergency procedures for a preventive exercise program.

SLO
Identify emergency drugs which should be available during exercise testing and demonstrate ability to assist a physician during an emergency situation.

EXERCISE LEADERSHIP

GO
The fitness instructor will demonstrate competence in the administrative concerns of effective exercise leadership.

A. Describe an organizational plan for facilities equipment, and consumable supplies for an exercise program.
B. Describe considerations involved in scheduling events and staff.
C. Identify factors related to efficient data entry, storage, retrieval and feedback to participants, physicians and other involved persons.
D. Implement evaluation procedures of testing, exercise, and patient education programs.

SLO
Identify and describe possible causes and intervention techniques regarding common orthopedic problems associated with physical activity and adaptations required in exercise prescription: include myositis ossificans, shin splints, tennis elbow, bursitis, stress fracture, lordosis, tendonitis, contusion and osteoporosis.

HUMAN BEHAVIOR/PSYCHOLOGY

SLO
Describe psychologic and physiologic responses to stressful situations. Discuss stress management techniques to elicit relaxation.

SLO
Define or describe each of the following terms in relation to the management of an exercise program: aggression, hostility, denial, identification, operant conditioning, rapport, anxiety, empathy, fear, rationalization, relaxation, euphoria, depression, and rejection.

HUMAN DEVELOPMENT/AGING

SLO
List the differences in conditioning older vs. younger participants.

SLO

Describe leadership techniques which might need to be adjusted because of vision or hearing impairments of participants.

SLO

Describe the modification of exercise programming as it relates to the aging process (childhood through the older adult).

FUNCTIONAL ANATOMY AND KINESIOLOGY

GO

The fitness instructor will demonstrate an understanding of general anatomy and kinesiology.

SLO

Given anatomic models or diagrams the fitness instructor will:

A. Identify the major bones, muscle groups, and diarthradial joints of the human body; describe how each affects the joint range of motion.
B. Identify the cardiovascular anatomy specifically, chambers, valves, vessels and the conduction system.

SLO

Describe differences in the mechanics of human locomotion in walking, jogging, running, lifting weights and carrying or moving objects.

SLO

Define and describe the practical application of the following: center of gravity, base of support, heel strike, dissipation of force, rebound.

SLO

Describe and demonstrate exercises for specific muscle groups.

HEALTH FITNESS DIRECTOR: BEHAVIORAL OBJECTIVES

PROGRAM ADMINISTRATION

GO

The health fitness director will understand the role of administration as a means of program facilitation.

SLO

Describe a management plan for staff resource development, facilities management, and financial planning.

SLO

Describe the value of cost/benefit, value analysis and evaluation criteria in the decision making process.

SLO

Discuss the advantages and/or disadvantages of centralized, decentralized and matrix project management.

SLO

Identify a personnel management program, including staff growth and development, evaluation, and procedures for professional advancement.

SLO
Describe effective planning, resource estimation and scheduling for both short and long-term goals.

SLO
Demonstrate and describe a management-by-objective approach to specific projects (i.e., increase facility utilization, facility expansion, marketing).

SLO
Describe personnel time management techniques for effective administration.

SLO
Describe a technique for clientele tracking, billing and personnel utilization.

SLO
Describe and understand the role of external resources in short-term and long-term program planning.

SLO
Describe skills involved in interviewing candidates, writing job descriptions and contracting for services.

SLO
Describe the steps in developing, evaluating, revising, and updating capital and operating budgets.

SLO
Describe the process of facility design and equipment selection purchase.

SLO
Demonstrate an understanding of public relations strategies.

SLO
Identify the steps in development, implementation and evaluation of a marketing plan.

SLO
Describe the components of an advertising program including objectives, resources and techniques.

SLO
Demonstrate effective skills and techniques for communications, public speaking, and use of audiovisuals for presentations to groups and individuals.

SLO
Diagram and explain an organizational chart and show the staff relationships between a health fitness director, governing body, medical advisor, participant's personal physician, staff and participants.

SLO
Identify and explain operating policies for preventive exercise programs including data analysis and reporting, reimbursement of service fees, confidentiality of records, relationships between program and

referring physicians, continuing education of participant and family, legal liability, and accident or injury reporting.

SLO
Explain the legal concepts of tort, negligence, contributory negligence, liability, standards of care, consent, contract, confidentiality, and malpractice.

SLO
Design and coordinate research efforts which may evolve from testing, exercise, or educational programs.

SLO
Interpret applied research in the areas of testing, exercise, and educational programs in order to update programs and stay current with the state-of-the-art.

EXERCISE PHYSIOLOGY

GO
The health fitness director will demonstrate a knowledge and a theoretical understanding of exercise physiology.

SLO
Demonstrate an understanding of the relationship between muscle structure and function.

A. Describe the structure of muscle fiber.
B. Describe the functional characteristics of fast and slow twitch fibers.
C. Explain contraction of muscle in terms of the sliding filament theory.
D. Explain twitch, summation, and tetanus in terms of muscle contraction.
E. Explain the concepts of muscle fatigue under specific conditions of task, intensity, and duration of exercise.

SLO
Demonstrate an understanding of the metabolic and cardiorespiratory response to exercise and explain their interrelationships.

A. Describe and explain the mechanisms by which heart rate (HR), stroke volume (SV), cardiac output ($\dot{Q}$), arteriovenous O_2 difference ($a - \bar{v}O_2$ diff), O_2 uptake ($\dot{V}O_2$), systolic, diastolic blood pressure (SBP, DBP), minute ventilation ($\dot{V}_E$), tidal volume (V_T), breathing frequency (f), and respiratory exchange ratio (RER) change with increasing work intensities in conditioned and unconditioned adults of varying ages (some physiologic mechanisms may not be known).
B. Explain the contribution of aerobic and anaerobic metabolism to the total energy cost of exercise at maximum and at different intensities of exercise.
C. Explain the adaptations and characteristics which differentiate

the conditioned from the unconditioned adult, in particular cardiorespiratory and musculoskeletal changes.

D. Explain the concept of the reversibility of conditioning.

EMERGENCY PROCEDURES

GO

The health fitness director will demonstrate competence in the use, maintenance, and updating of appropriate emergency equipment, supplies, and evacuation plans.

SLO

Teach the principles and techniques used in cardiopulmonary resuscitation.

SLO

Demonstrate the emergency procedures, equipment, and materials needed during exercise testing, fitness evaluations, and exercise sessions.

SLO

Discuss the individual responsibility and legal implications related to emergency care.

SLO

Design and update emergency procedures for a preventive exercise program.

SLO

Identify emergency drugs which should be available during exercise testing and demonstrate ability to assist a physician during an emergency situation.

PATHOPHYSIOLOGY

GO

The health fitness director will understand the interrelationship between different diseases or conditions and physical activity.

SLO

Explain the process of atherosclerosis.

SLO

Describe how lifestyle factors and heredity influence lipoprotein profiles.

SLO

Explain the causes of myocardial ischemia and infarction.

SLO

Explain the causes of hypertension, obesity, diabetes, chronic obstructive and restrictive pulmonary diseases, arthritis and gout.

SLO

Identify and explain the effects of the above diseases or conditions on cardiorespiratory and metabolic function at rest and during exercise.

SLO

Explain the risk factor concept of coronary artery disease (CAD) and the influence of heredity and lifestyle upon the development of CAD.

SLO

Explain the use and value of the results of the exercise test and fitness evaluation for various populations.

SLO

Identify and explain the mechanisms by which exercise may contribute to preventing the above diseases.

SLO

Describe muscular, cardiorespiratory, and metabolic responses to exercise following a decrease in physical activity, bed rest, or casting of a limb for a period of 1 month.

SLO

Explain the causes and mechanisms of chronic obstructive pulmonary disease (COPD), exercised induced asthma, and chronic asthma.

SLO

Identify current drugs from each of the following classes. Explain the principal action, and list its major side-effects,

A. Antianginal
B. Antiarrhythmic
C. Antihypertensive
D. Bronchodilators
E. Hypoglycemics
F. Psychologic stimulants

ELECTROCARDIOGRAPHY

GO

The health fitness director will understand the basic electrocardiographic responses at rest and during exercise testing and conditioning.

SLO

Identify ECG evidence of myocardial infarction, ST depression, ST elevation, significant Q waves, bradycardia, tachycardia, AV blocks, ventricular arrhythmias, atrial arrhythmias, ventricular hypertrophy, and bundle branch blocks.

SLO

Explain possible causes of a false positive or false negative exercise test. Discuss methods of avoiding a false positive/negative exercise test.

HUMAN BEHAVIOR/PSYCHOLOGY

GO

The health fitness program director will demonstrate an understanding of basic principles of human behavior and group dynamics to include communication, motivation, and factors which influence behavior over time.

SLO
Recognize the behavior changes associated with the initiation of an exercise program.

SLO
Understand the factors supporting or inhibiting these changes.

SLO
Identify and explain factors influencing the effectiveness of communication.

GO
The health fitness director will demonstrate an understanding of the effect of psychologic stress on physiologic systems.

SLO
Identify the effects of psychological stress on the following systems—cardiovascular, pulmonary, circulatory, and neuromuscular.

HUMAN DEVELOPMENT/AGING

GO
The health fitness director will demonstrate an understanding of the effect of the aging process on the structure and function of the human organism at rest, during exercise, and after conditioning.

SLO
Identify and explain the cardiorespiratory response to exercise in persons of advancing age, in adolescents, and in children.

SLO
Explain the differences in conditioning of older compared to younger participants, with regard to strength, functional capacity, mechanical efficiency, reaction and movement time, flexibility, coordination, and tolerance to heat and cold.

SLO
Describe common orthopedic and cardiorespiratory problems of older participants and explain how modification of exercise can reduce their aggravation.

FUNCTIONAL ANATOMY AND KINESIOLOGY

GO
The health fitness director will demonstrate knowledge of human functional anatomy.

SLO
Explain how bio-mechanical factors influence performance with implications for the selection and conduct of physical exercise.

SLO
Analyze and evaluate varieties of exercises and movements to predict their influence upon structure, growth, efficiency, and health.

INTERNSHIP

In order to qualify as a health fitness director, an internship or period of practical experience of at least 1 year is required. The internship should be under the supervision of a certified exercise program director and a physician and provide opportunities to obtain competencies in administration, program leadership, laboratory procedures, and exercise prescription. It is assumed that the preceptor of the internship will work closely with the prospective health fitness program director. In addition to the opportunity to demonstrate proficiency, oral and written examinations are an integral part of the learning experience.

PREVENTIVE AND REHABILITATIVE EXERCISE SPECIALIST

Exercise appears to have an appropriate and accepted role in preventive and rehabilitative medical programs. The unique competency of the preventive and rehabilitative exercise specialist is the ability to lead exercise for persons with medical limitations, especially cardiorespiratory and related diseases, as well as to lead exercise for healthy asymptomatic populations. The exercise specialist, in conjunction with the program director or physician, must be able to design an exercise prescription based on the results of an exercise test, evaluate participants' responses to exercise and conditioning, assist in the education of patients, and interact and communicate effectively with the physician, program director, exercise test technologist, program participants, and with the community at large.

The exercise specialist must demonstrate the competencies required of the exercise test technologist and health fitness instructor, as specified elsewhere in this chapter. Curricula that enhance the preparation for the position of exercise specialist include, but are not limited to, exercise physiology and the allied health professions. An internship of at least 6 months, (approximately 800 hours) is required before applying for certification. This internship should be under the direction of a physician or rehabilitative exercise program director and primarily include a variety of experiences including exercise testing, prescription, and supervision of individual and group exercise programs for participants with medically diagnosed disease or limitations, particularly cardiorespiratory disease.

An exercise specialist in activity programs for prevention and rehabilitation of individuals with medical or physical limitations is required to apply scientific principles of conditioning and motivating techniques for establishing a healthy lifestyle.

In all appropriately supervised exercise sessions the goal should be to offer activities that will improve the participant's functional capacity. Exposure to and instruction in a variety of activities is encouraged. Positive attitudes toward work and leisure as well as positive physical benefits are desired outcomes.

Certain knowledge about leading physical activity can be learned. The exercise leader must be able to evaluate the physiologic effects of exercise and possess the ability to incorporate suitable and innovative activities for each individual. Preventive and rehabilitative programs require that participants not only establish, but adhere to long-range commitments to regular physical activity in order to maintain optimal levels of fitness. Programs need to include motivational, counseling, teaching, and behavior modification techniques to emphasize current and valid health information and promote life-style changes. Knowledge of the scientific principles of exercise and conditioning, and the ability to design safe, appropriate, and enjoyable individualized exercise prescriptions, particularly for persons with cardiac disease, are the primary objectives for a well-prepared and competent exercise specialist.

BEHAVIORAL OBJECTIVES

The exercise specialist, in addition to meeting the behavioral objectives outlined for the exercise test technologist and health fitness instructor will demonstrate competence in exercise prescription and leadership in preventive and rehabilitative exercise programs for participants with medically diagnosed disease or limitations, in particular, those with cardiac disease.

REHABILITATIVE EXERCISE PRESCRIPTION

GO

The exercise specialist will demonstrate an understanding of the implications of exercise for persons with observed coronary heart disease (CHD) risk factors and for patients with established cardiovascular, respiratory, metabolic, or orthopedic disorders and demonstrate competence in executing individualized exercise prescription.

SLO

Given sufficient medical information and the results of an exercise test, the exercise specialist will:

A. Prior to the implementation of the exercise program use the test data for prescribing appropriate exercise, including intensity, duration, frequency, progression, type of physical activity, and whether exercise is to be supervised or unsupervised;
B. Modify type of physical activity, intensity, duration, progression,

(temporarily or permanently) according to the current health status of the participant (e.g., immediate post-surgical or MI, common metabolic, cardiorespiratory, and orthopedic conditions);

C. Demonstrate the use of a goniometer in the assessment of mobility and flexibility of major joints;
D. Identify warm-up and cool-down phenomena with specific reference to angina and ischemic ECG changes;
E. Describe the inherent physiologic phenomena which exclude certain types of exercises from a rehabilitative exercise program;
F. Describe the physiologic consequences of certain postural changes, especially during the period following vigorous activity;
G. Describe appropriate exercises to reduce the deconditioning effects of bed rest and appropriate methods of progressing exercise levels to return hospitalized patients to daily living tasks;
H. Describe the precautions taken before, during, and after physical activity at high altitude and at different ambient temperatures and humidities with specific reference to the patient with cardiorespiratory limitations;
I. Describe contraindications to exercise or inappropriate exercise responses which would be an indication for termination of the exercise session according to the current health status of the participant (e.g., early post-surgical or MI, common metabolic, cardiorespiratory, orthopedic conditions);

SLO
Given a clinical case study, devise supervised exercise programs for the first 6 weeks after discharge from the hospital and then for the 3 months following.

SLO
Discuss common modifications in exercise programming for the patient with obstructive pulmonary disease, asthma and restrictive pulmonary disease.

REHABILITATIVE EXERCISE LEADERSHIP

GO
The exercise specialist will demonstrate competence in leading and supervising physical activity in rehabilitative exercise programs.

SLO
Given a case study and subject(s) primarily with cardiac disease, lead appropriate exercises based on a prescription executed from the exercise test and other clinical and behavioral data.

GO
The exercise specialist will demonstrate competence in the administrative concerns of effective exercise leadership.

SLO
Describe considerations involved in scheduling rehabilitative program events and in making staff assignments.

SLO

Implement evaluation procedures of laboratory testing, exercise conditioning and patient education programs.

REHABILITATIVE EMERGENCY PROCEDURES

GO

The exercise specialist will demonstrate competence in responding with the appropriate emergency procedures to situations in rehabilitative settings which might arise prior, during, and after exercise.

SLO

Diagram an emergency response system and discuss minimum standards for equipment and personnel required in settings for rehabilitative exercise programs.

REHABILITATIVE EXERCISE TESTING

GO

The exercise specialist will demonstrate competence in the interpretation of the exercise test for a rehabilitation program patient relative to the assessment of functional capacity, and using these data, provide objective recommendations regarding the patient's ability to engage in physical conditioning, return to work and to perform select physical activities (e.g. automobile driving, stair climbing, sexual activity) following a cardiovascular event.

REHABILITATIVE EXERCISE PHYSIOLOGY

GO

The exercise specialist will demonstrate an understanding of exercise physiology.

SLO

Describe the implications of aerobic and anaerobic metabolic demands in various exercises for rehabilitative clients.

SLO

Differentiate the function of the myocardium, the generation of the action potential, and major variants in pathways of electrical activation and repolarization in healthy vs coronary heart diseased persons.

SLO

Plot the following resting values and the normal values for increasing levels of exercise response to increasing intensity: heart rate (HR); stroke volume (SV); cardiac output ($\dot{Q}$); arteriovenous O_2 difference ($a-\bar{v}O_2$ diff); O_2 uptake ($\dot{V}O_2$) systolic and diastolic blood pressure (SBP, DBP); minute ventilation ($\dot{V}_E$); tidal volume (V_T); breathing frequency (f). Indicate how certain of the preceding values may differ for the rehabilitative client.

SLO

Explain the difference in the cardiorespiratory responses to static (isometric) exercise compared with dynamic (isotonic) exercise; include possible hazards of isometric exercise for low-functional capacity adults or patients with cardiovascular disease.

SLO
Explain the specificity of conditioning and the physiologic differences among cardiorespiratory, muscular endurance, and muscular strength conditioning; include the mechanism by which the functional capacity and skeletal muscle hypertrophy increase during a conditioning program.

SLO
Describe and design acceptable laboratory and field exercise test protocols from which functional capacity or VO_2 max determinations or estimations may be obtained in low-functional capacity subjects and patients with cardiovascular disease.

SLO
Define the detrimental effects of bed rest and how appropriate physical activities might be used to offset, somewhat, the physiologic effects of bedrest in hospitalized patients and those undergoing an early post-hospital rehabilitation program.

SLO
Compare the unique hemodynamic response of arm vs leg exercise and of static vs dynamic exercise.

REHABILITATIVE PATHOPHYSIOLOGY

GO
The exercise specialist will demonstrate an understanding of the cardiorespiratory and metabolic responses to increasing intensities of exercise in certain diseases and conditions.

SLO
Identify and describe the cardiorespiratory and metabolic responses in myocardial dysfunction and ischemia at rest and during exercise.

SLO
Identify the cardiorespiratory and metabolic responses in pulmonary disease at rest and during exercise.

SLO
Identify the signs and symptoms of peripheral vascular diseases and the effects different kinds of exercise may have on each.

SLO
Identify the metabolic responses and possible dysfunctions of a diabetic patient at rest and during exercise.

SLO
Explain the influence of exercise on weight reduction and hyperlipidemia.

SLO
Describe the effects of variation in ambient temperature, humidity, CO_2, and in altitude on functional capacity and the exercise prescription. Explain required adaptations to the exercise prescription when environmental extremes exist.

SLO
Describe the etiology of atherosclerosis.

SLO
Describe the implications, symptoms, and mechanisms of classical and vasospastic angina.

SLO
Discuss the pathophysiology of the healing myocardium.

SLO
List the common major symptoms of drug intolerance or toxicity in the following classes of medications. See Appendix B.

A. Antianginal (nitrates, beta blockers, etc.)
B. Antiarrhythmic
C. Anticoagulant
D. Antiplatelet aggregation
E. Lipid lowering drugs
F. Antihypertensive (diuretics, vasodilators, etc.)
G. Digitalis glycosides
H. Calcium channel blocking agents
I. Bronchodilators
J. Tranquilizers, antidepressants, and antianxiety drugs

SLO
List the major effects on physiologic responses and symptomatology, including ECG changes, of the above ten classes of drugs at rest and during exercise.

GO
The exercise specialist will demonstrate an understanding of various modalities applied in the medical diagnosis and therapeutic management of certain diseases.

SLO
Describe the purpose and utility of coronary angiography, thallium perfusion scanning and radionuclide cineangiography.

SLO
Describe percutaneous transluminal angioplasty.

SLO
Describe the use of streptokinase.

REHABILITATIVE ELECTROCARDIOGRAPHY

GO
The exercise specialist will demonstrate an understanding of the important electrocardiographic responses at rest and during exercise in healthy vs coronary artery diseased persons.

SLO
Explain possible causes of ischemia and various important cardiac arrhythmias. Explain the significance of their occurrence during rest, exercise, and recovery.

SLO
Identify the potentially hazardous arrhythmias or conduction defects that might be observed on the ECG at rest or during exercise and explain what procedures would be followed concerning a participant's care.

SLO
Identify the significance of important ECG abnormalities with special reference to exercise prescription and activity selection.

REHABILITATIVE HUMAN BEHAVIOR/PSYCHOLOGY

GO
The exercise specialist will demonstrate an understanding of basic behavioral psychological and group dynamics as they apply to crisis management, coping and lifestyle modifications in patients with certain chronic diseases.

SLO
Demonstrate an ability to apply the principles of lifestyle modification as these relate to participation in a rehabilitative exercise program.

SLO
Describe the general principles of crisis management and factors influencing coping and learning in illness states.

SLO
Recognize signs and symptoms of maladjustment/failure to cope during an illness crisis.

REHABILITATIVE INTERNSHIP

An internship of at least 6 months (800) hours is required, largely with cardiopulmonary disease patients in a rehabilitative setting, with specific experience to obtain competency in the following areas;

A. Conducting and administering of exercise tests;
B. Evaluating and interpreting of clinical data and exercise test results for the formulation of the exercise prescription;
C. Conducting exercise sessions including the demonstration of leadership, proper monitoring, enthusiasm and creativity;
D. Responding appropriately to complications during exercise testing and training;
E. Modifying the exercise prescription for patients with specific secondary limitations, beyond cardiopulmonary disease.

EXERCISE PROGRAM DIRECTOR

Exercise appears to have an appropriate and accepted role in both preventive and rehabilitative medical problems. As a result, there is an increasing demand for information about exercise testing, exercise prescription, and exercise programs by the medical and health-related professions and by the general public. In order to meet this demand an increasing number of qualified, specially trained exercise program directors are needed.

Because the persons who wish to become exercise program directors must have the knowledge and competencies of the exercise test technologist, health fitness instructor, health fitness director, and exercise specialist, it is probable that they already had much of the practical background necessary for the testing and physical conditioning portions of the program. To understand the medical and physiologic implications of exercise testing and the resulting exercise programs and to understand how and why certain activities are recommended or contraindicated more theoretical experience is needed. It is hoped that the majority of this knowledge will have been obtained during studies for an advanced degree in fields such as exercise physiology, physiology and medicine, or physical education.

Since the exercise program directors are responsible for (1) the inclusion of adequate exercise testing procedures, (2) accurate, individualized exercise prescriptions, and (3) careful supervision and leadership for safe, effective, and enjoyable exercise programs, they need the theoretical and practical backgrounds associated with certain aspects of medicine, physiology, physical education, and behavioral psychology. Thus, exercise program directors are unique specialists in that they must draw from a wide range of abilities, knowledge, and experience as they relate to exercise.

With this combination of theoretical knowledge and practical experiences, the program director should be capable of organizing and administering all types of programs in any situation. The program director should have the ability to plan and initiate new programs, as well as to reorganize and upgrade existing ones. The fact that one can work in programs for disease-limited patients and asymptomatic persons suggests that they possess the versatility, adaptability, and breadth of knowledge and experience necessary for certification as a preventive and rehabilitative exercise program director. The same may not be the case for those who have worked only with athletes or children. It is for this reason that there is so much emphasis on the preventive and rehabilitative aspects of exercise.

The exact role of the program director depends on factors such as personal interest, the size of the program, and the type of people who will be tested and exercised. If the program is small, then the program director may be involved in the collection and analysis of data obtained during exercise testing or the supervision and leadership of the actual exercise programs. If the program is relatively large, then the duties may be primarily administrative and related to the actual prescription of the activity program in close cooperation with the physician. The program director's duties will also include the training, continuing education, and supervision of the other personnel, i.e., the exercise test technologists, health fitness instructors, and exercise specialists. The program director should understand the basic aspects of behavior modification, emergency procedures, particular problems of special groups of patients, and program administration.

An exercise program director must also work with and communicate with the public, those persons who are tested and who are exercised, and with physicians and health professionals, i.e., with people who have varying degrees of knowledge and sophistication regarding the medical, physiologic, psychologic, and educational aspects of exercise programs. Because of this, the program director should understand and be able to explain and discuss both the theoretical and practical aspects of exercise and conditioning with each of these various groups of people. This ability to communicate is especially important since people in exercise programs should be able not only to improve physical condition, but also to acquire a certain degree of autonomy in that improvement. For example, participants cannot always remain in a supervised controlled exercise program. For this reason, a program of continuing education is important so that the participants can continue to lead active, more healthful lives when they no longer desire or are not able to continue in a supervised program.

In special programs for middle-aged or older persons, for persons who have a high risk of developing a disease such as coronary heart disease, or for those who already have specific medical problems, the program director must understand the medical and physiologic implications of the medical history of these patients and provide for any special needs related to the testing, prescription, and supervision of exercises. In doing this, the program director is expected to maintain a close working relationship with appropriate medical specialists. In such cases where the knowledge and experience necessary to work with these special groups are inadequate and were not integral parts of their educational background, program directors are expected to study and learn more about any special aspects of a particular medical or physiologic problem by means of special courses or symposia, by reading scientific articles and books, by discussions with knowledgeable persons, and by conducting research. In other words, exercise program directors should be "life-time students" who continuously strive to improve the level of competency within their speciality.

Professional study and cooperation of the program director with physicians, physiologists, physical educators, and other health personnel are basic to the optimal realization of the health benefits from physical activity programs. This type of team work is especially needed if the benefits from these programs are to be made available to large segments of the public. The program director can and should be a major factor in the success of such a program.

BEHAVIORAL OBJECTIVES

The exercise program director, in addition to meeting the behavioral objectives outlined for the exercise specialist, health fitness instructor, exercise test technologist, and the health fitness director, will demonstrate competency in designing, implementing, and administering preventive and rehabilitative exercise programs and educating the staff and members of the community about physical activity in programs of disease prevention and rehabilitation. This includes the following behavioral objectives.

PROGRAM ADMINISTRATION

GO

The exercise program director will understand the role of administration as a means of program facilitation.

SLO

Diagram and explain an organizational chart and show the staff relationships between an exercise program director, governing body, exercise specialist, exercise test technologist, fitness instructor, medical advisor, participants's personal physician, and participants.

SLO

Identify and explain operating policies for preventive and rehabilitative exercise programs including data analysis and reporting, reimbursement of service fees, confidentiality of records, relationships between program and referring physicians, continuing education of staff, continuing education of participant and family, legal liability, accident or injury reporting, emergency procedures, and hiring and firing.

SLO

Describe program direction evaluation.

SLO
Identify safety requirements and equipment.

SLO
Describe and explain strategies of public and human relations, including techniques for informing members of the community about physical activity programs of prevention and rehabilitation.

EMERGENCY PROCEDURES

(See Behavioral Objectives—Health Fitness Director)

FUNCTIONAL ANATOMY

(See Behavioral Objectives—Health Fitness Director)

EXERCISE PHYSIOLOGY

GO
The exercise program director will demonstrate a knowledge and a theoretical understanding of exercise physiology.

SLO
Demonstrate an understanding of the basic electrophysiology of cardiac muscle by explaining the properties of cardiac muscle and the normal and abnormal conduction patterns of the propagation of action potentials across the myocardium.

SLO
Demonstrate an understanding of the metabolic and cardiorespiratory response to exercise and explain their interrelationships.

A. Describe the physiologic changes which would lower myocardial oxygen consumption for a given submaximal exercise intensity following a physical conditioning program.
B. Describe the biochemistry of muscle fatigue under specific conditions of task, intensity, and duration of exercise.

PATHOPHYSIOLOGY

GO
The exercise program director will demonstrate an understanding of the interrelationship between different disease states or conditions and physical activity.

SLO
Explain the process of atherosclerosis including current hypotheses regarding onset, rate of progression and the role of lipoprotein phenotypes.

SLO
Demonstrate an understanding of lipoprotein classifications.

SLO
Discuss the similarities and differences of the signs and symptoms in the pulmonary versus cardiac patient during exercise testing and exercise training.

SLO

Explain the diagnostic and prognostic value of the results of the graded exercise test for various populations.

SLO

Explain the diagnostic and prognostic value of the low level predischarge exercise test versus the symptom-limited test and the appropriateness for use with CHD patients.

SLO

Identify and explain the mechanisms by which exercise may contribute to preventing the above diseases and rehabilitating individuals with the above diseases.

SLO

Name at least one drug from each of the following classes, explain the mechanism of its principal action, and list its major side-effects, including ECG changes at rest and during exercise. See Appendix B.

A. Antianginal
B. Antiarrhythmic
C. Anticoagulant
D. Antiplatelet aggregation
E. Lipid lowering drugs
F. Antihypertensive
G. Digitalis glycosides
H. Calcium channel blocking agents
I. Bronchodilators
J. Hypoglycemics
K. "Mood" elevators; stimulants

GO

The program director will demonstrate an understanding of the various diagnostic and treatment modalities currently used in the management of coronary heart disease, including myocardial infarction, coronary bypass surgery, and valvular heart disease.

SLO

Describe coronary angiography, Thallium scanning, and gated pool studies including the type of information obtained, sensitivity and specificity, and associated risks.

SLO

Describe percutaneous transluminal angioplasty as an alternative to medical management or coronary artery bypass surgery in CHD. Demonstrate an understanding of the indications for percutaneous transluminal angioplasty in different subsets of CHD patients versus coronary bypass surgery or management with medications.

SLO

Describe the use of streptokinase infusion in acute myocardial infarction.

ELECTROCARDIOGRAPHY

GO

The program director will understand electrocardiographic responses at rest and during exercise testing and conditioning.

SLO

Explain the functioning of cardiac pacemakers and the precautions to be taken by individuals with pacemakers.

SLO

Explain the diagnostic and prognostic value of the occurrence of ischemic or arrhythmic responses at rest, during exercise, or during recovery in asymptomatic participants, patients with stable CHD and those at different stages after coronary bypass surgery or myocardial infarction, and patients following valvular heart surgery or other types of open heart surgical procedures.

HUMAN BEHAVIOR/PSYCHOLOGY

GO

The exercise program director will understand the role of the exercise rehabilitation program in screening, identification and referral of patients with psychologic disorders.

SLO

Describe community resources for psychologic support and behavior modification and outline an example of a referral system.

HUMAN DEVELOPMENT/AGING

(See Behavioral Objectives—Health Fitness Director)

INTERNSHIP

An internship or period of practical experience of at least 2 years is required.

APPENDIX A

Informed Consent for an Exercise Test (Sample)

1. *Explanation of the Exercise Test*

You will perform an exercise test on a cycle ergometer or a motor-driven treadmill. The exercise intensity will begin at a level you can easily accomplish and will be advanced in stages, depending on your fitness level. We may stop the test at any time because of signs of fatigue or you may stop when you wish because of personal feelings of fatigue or discomfort.

2. *Risks and Discomforts*

There exists the possibility of certain changes occurring during the test. They include abnormal blood pressure, fainting, disorder of heart beat, and in rare instances, heart attack or death. Every effort will be made to minimize these through the preliminary examination and by observations during testing. Emergency equipment and trained personnel are available to deal with unusual situations which may arise.

3. *Benefits to be Expected*

The results obtained from the exercise test may assist in the diagnosis of your illness or in evaluating what type of physical activities you might engage with no or low hazards.

4. *Inquiries*

Any questions about the procedures used in the exercise test or in the estimation of functional capacity are encouraged. If you have any doubts or questions, please ask us for further explanations.

5. *Freedom of Consent*

Your permission to perform this exercise test is voluntary. You are free to deny consent if you so desire.

I have read this form and I understand the test procedures that I will perform. I consent to participate in this test.

____
Signature of Patient

____________________ ____________________________
Date Witness

Questions:____

____

Response: ____

____

Physician signature: optional.

When test is for purpose other than diagnosis or prescription, e.g. experimental interest, this should be indicated on the Informed Consent Form.

Policy on Human Subjects for Research is available on request from ACSM.

APPENDIX B

Pharmacologic Agents Which May Be Encountered in Cardiac Patients

Appendix B Pharmacologic Agents Which May Be Encountered in Cardiac Patients

Drugs	Effect[a]				
	Exercise Performance	*H.R.*	*B.P.*	*Effect on ECG*	*Effect on Exercise ECG*
I. ANTIANGINAL					
A. NITRATES/OTHERS					May delay onset of ischemic response
Nitroglycerin (Nitrobid)					
Isosorbide Dinitrate (Isordil) (Sorbitrate)	↑[b,e]	↑	↓		
Erythrityle Tetranitrate (Cardilate)					
Pentaerythritol Tetranitrate (Peritrate)					
Nitroglycerin Patch (Nitro-Dur)					
Dypyridamole (Persantine)					
B. BETA BLOCKERS				U waves may become prominent due to bradycardia	May delay onset of ischemic response
Pindolol (Visken)					
Propranolol (Inderal)	↑[b]↓	↓	↓		
Metoprolol Tartrate (Lopressor)					
Nadolol (Corgard)					
Atenolol (Tenormin)					
Timolol (Blocadren)					
C. CALCIUM CHANNEL BLOCKERS					May delay onset of ischemia
Nifedipine (Procardia)	↑[b]	↑[c]	↓		
Verapamil (Isoptin) (Calan)	↑[b]	↓[d]	↓		
Diltiazem (Cardizem)	↑[b]		↓		
II. ANTIHYPERTENSIVE					
A. DIURETICS				Prolongs QT interval, accentuates U waves if hypokalemic	May cause False–Positive if hypokalemic
Hydrochlorothiazide IEsidrix)					
Chlorothiazide (Diuril)			↓		
Methylchothiazide (Enduron)					
Furosemide (Lasix)					

B. POTASSIUM SPARING DIURETICS Triamterene (Dyrenium) Spironolactone (Aldactone)			↓	Tall T waves and other ECG changes if hyperkalemic	
C. VASODILATOR Hydralazine (Apresoline) Prazosin (Minipress)		↑	↓		
D. CENTRAL NERVOUS SYSTEM ACTIVE Reserpine (Serpasil) Guanethidine (Ismelin) Clonidine (Catapres)		↓	↓		
E. BETA BLOCKERS (SEE IB.)					
F. CALCIUM CHANNEL BLOCKERS (SEE IC.)					
G. OTHER Captopril (Capoten)	↑[e]		↓		
III. ANTIARRHYTHMICS (TACHYARRHYTHMIAS) A. DRUGS WITH MULTIPLE ACTIONS Phenytoin (Dilantin) Lidocaine (Xylocaine) Procainamide (Pronestyl) Quinidine Gluconate or Sulfate (Quinaglute) (Quinidine) Disopyramide Phosphate (Norpace)				U wave changes, widening of QRS, QT changes	Quinidine and Quinaglute may delay onset of ischemic response
B. BETA BLOCKERS (SEE IB.)					
C. CALCIUM CHANNEL BLOCKERS (SEE IC.)					

[a]Effects apply to all drugs in the group unless otherwise noted. Absence of information on an effect for a given drug indicates no known significant effect.
[b]If the patient has angina.
[c]Nifedipine
[d]Verapamil
[e]If the patient has heart failure.

Appendix B Pharmacologic Agents Which May Be Encountered in Cardiac Patients *CONTINUED*

	Effect[a]				
Drugs	*Exercise Performance*	*H.R.*	*B.P.*	*Effect on ECG*	*Effect on Exercise ECG*
D. DIGITALIS PREPARATIONS Digitoxin (Crystodigin) Digoxin (Lanoxin)	↑[b]	↑ With toxicity or may ↓ if blocks A-V node[c]		May produce ST-depression accentuated with exercise	May produce ST-depression accentuated with exercise
(BRADYARRHYTHMIAS) A. PARASYMPATHETIC BLOCKERS Atropine		↑			
B. SYMPATHOMIMETICS					
Isoproterenol (Isuprel)		↑	↑	May cause ectopic beats	May cause ectopic beats
Epinephrine				May cause ectopic beats	May cause ectopic beats
IV. ANTI-CONGESTIVE HEART FAILURE A. DIURETICS (SEE IIA.)					
B. DIGITALIS (SEE IIID.)					
V. BRONCHODILATORS					
Aminophylline	↑ ↓	↑	↑ ↓	May cause ectopic beats	May cause ectopic beats
Theophylline	↑ ↓	↑	↑ ↓	May cause ectopic beats	May cause ectopic beats
Albuterol (Ventolin) (Proventil)	↑ ↓	↑	↑ ↓	May cause ectopic beats	Ectopic beats may lower threshold to angina
Isoproterenol (Isuprel)	↑	↑	↑ (Isoproterenol)		Ectopic beats may lower threshold to angina

VI. ANTI-LIPEMIC				
Gemfibrozil (Lopid)				
Clofibrate (Atromid-S)	↑ (Choloxin)	↑ (Choloxin)	May cause ectopic beats (Clofibrate)	May cause ectopic beats (Clofibrate)
Dextrothyroxine (Choloxin)			May cause ectopic beats, tachycardia or evidence of ischemia (Dextro-thyroxine)	May cause ectopic beats, tachycardia or evidence of ischemia (Dextrothyroxine)
Colestipol (Colestid)		↓ (Niacin)	Prolonged QT (Probucol)	
Probuco (Lorelco)				
Niacin (Nicolar)				
Cholestyramine (Questran)				
VII. ANTICOAGULANTS				
A Heparin				
VIII. ANTI GOUT				
Sulfinpyrazone (Anturane)				
IX. ANTI PSYCHONEUROSIS				
A. TRANQUILIZERS			T & U wave changes	May cause False-Positive or False-Negative
Phenothiazines	↑	↓		
B. ANTIDEPRESSANTS				
Imipramine (Tofranil)	↑	↓	May cause arrhythmias	May cause False-Positive
Amitriptyline (Elavil)				
C. ANTIANXIETY				
Lithium	↓	↓	ST-T wave changes	May cause False-Positive
Diazepam (Valium)	(Diazepam)	(Diazepam)		

[a]Effects apply to all drugs in the group unless otherwise noted. Absence of information on an effect for a given drug indicates no known significant effect.
[b]If the patient has heart failure.
[c]With atrial fibrillation.

Appendix B Pharmacologic Agents Which May Be Encountered in Cardiac Patients *CONTINUED*

	Effect[a]				
Drugs	*Exercise Performance*	*H.R.*	*B.P.*	*Effect on ECG*	*Effect on Exercise ECG*
X. HYPOGLYCEMIC					
A. ORAL					
Acetohexamide (Dymelor)					
Chlorpropamide (Diabinese)					
Tolazamide (Tolinase)					
Tolbutamide (Orinase)					
B. PARENTERAL					
Insulin					
XI. OTHERS					
Nicotine					
Antihistamines with Decongestants		↑	↑		
Thyroid Drugs					
Alcohol					

[a]Effects apply to all drugs in the group unless otherwise noted. Absence of information on an effect for a given drug indicates no known significant effect.

APPENDIX C

Informed Consent for a Cardiac Outpatient Rehabilitation Program

1. Explanation of Outpatient Cardiac Rehabilitation Program

You will be placed in a rehabilitation program that will include physical exercises. The levels of exercise which you will undertake will be based on your cardiovascular response to an initial exercise test. You will be given explicit instructions regarding the amount and kind of regular exercise you should do. Organized exercise sessions will be available on a regularly scheduled basis. Your exercise sessions may be adjusted by the exercise specialist in consultation with the exercise program director and physician depending on your progress. You will be given the opportunity for re-evaluation with a graded exercise test __________months after the initiation of the rehabilitation program, and __________thereafter. Other retests may be recommended as needed.

2. Monitoring

Your pre-exercise blood pressure will be monitored as required. You will monitor your own pulse rate before, during, and after each exercise session. In addition, ECG monitoring of your exercise prescription will be performed on a __________ basis or as needed.

3. Risks and Discomforts

There exists the possibility of certain changes occurring during the exercise sessions. These include abnormal blood pressure, fainting, disorders of heart beat, and in rare instances heart attack or death. Every effort will be made to minimize those risks by the preliminary examination and by observations during exercise. Emergency equipment and trained personnel are available to deal with unusual situations which may arise.

4. Benefits To Be Expected

Participation in the rehabilitation program may not benefit you directly in any way. The results obtained may help in evaluating in what types of activities you may engage safely in your daily life. No assurance can be given that the rehabilitation program will increase your functional capacity although widespread experience indicates that improvement is usually achieved.

5. Responsibility of the Participant

To gain expected benefits you must give priority to regular attendance and adherence to prescribed amounts of intensity, duration, frequency, progression, and type of activity.

To achieve the best possible preventive health care: DO NOT:

A. Withhold any information pertinent to symptoms from the exercise specialist, nurse, physician, exercise program director, or other professional personnel.
B. Exceed your target heart rate.
C. Exercise when you do not feel well.
D. Exercise within 2 hours after eating.
E. Exercise after drinking alcoholic beverages.
F. Use extremely hot water during showering after exercise (stay out of sauna, steam bath, and similar extreme temperatures).

DO:

A. Report any unusual symptom which you experience before, during, or after exercise, or you notice in an exercising colleague.
B. Check in with the exercise specialist after showering/dressing before leaving the site. If you plan to use other facilities at the site, please indicate that you will be doing so to the exercise specialist. At that time you must accept responsibility for yourself, and exercise at your own risk.

6. Use of Medical Records

The information which is obtained during exercise testing and while I am a participant in the Cardiac Rehabilitation program will be treated as privileged and confidential. It is not to be released or revealed to any person except my referring physician without my written consent. The information obtained however, may be used for statistical analysis or scientific purpose with my right to privacy retained.

7. Inquiries

Any questions about the rehabilitation program are welcome. If you have doubts or questions, please ask us for further explanation.

8. Freedom of Consent

Your permission to engage in this Rehabilitation Program is voluntary. You are free to deny any consent if you so desire, both now and at any point in the program.

I acknowledge that I have read this form in its entirety or it has been read to me, and that I understand the Rehabilitation Program in which I will be engaged. I accept the rules and regulations set forth. I consent to participate in this Rehabilitation Program.

Questions: ____

____

____

____

____

Response: ____

____

____

____

____

____
Signature of Patient

______________________ ______________________________
Date Witness

APPENDIX D

Metabolic Calculations

Introduction

The rate of energy expenditure ($\dot{E}$) during exercise is often assessed through indirect calorimetry by the measurement of the rate of oxygen consumption ($\dot{V}O_2$). Clinically this measurement often is not available. Therefore, there is a need for simple and reasonably accurate estimates of $\dot{E}$ (e.g., $\dot{V}O_2$, METs) during steady state exercise. Considerable confusion arises over terminology.* The physical functions of force, work and power which are described below relate to the mechanical aspects of ergometry (the measurement of "work"). These mechanical aspects of ergometry have metabolic equivalents. We are primarily concerned with the metabolic equivalents, since they relate to "how much" or "how hard" the exercise is in biologic terms. The "load" applied is the mechanical element that stimulates an increased metabolism (the metabolic equivalent) during exercise. The purpose of the equations which follow is to relate mechanical measures of work rates to their metabolic equivalents and vice versa. These estimates are appropriate for general clinical usage when using standard ergometric devices but may have limited applications in other settings.

---

*The American College of Sports Medicine has published definitions of terms and units used in sports science. See *Medicine and Science in Sports and Exercise,* Information for authors revised June, 1984.

Definitions

The terms presented below can be expressed in many different units. Mechanical or non-metabolic measurements are expressed in units of the Système International d'Unités (SI) in scientific writing. Although these units may not be the most understandable units clinically, they are prefered. SI units are starred (*) in the text.

1. Force (F): An accelerating mass ($F = m \times a$, where m = mass and a = acceleration). A weight is a force. It is a mass undergoing gravitational acceleration. Typical units of weight are pounds (lbs), newtons (N)*, kiloponds (kp), kilograms (kg). (A kilogram is really a unit of mass, but in common usage, it is used as a weight). Kilograms will be used throughout this section both for body weight and for the amount of weight applied to an ergometer. Strictly, one kilopond = one kilogram (mass) undergoing unit gravitational acceleration. Thus, we typically write "1 kg = 1 kp" and they are often used interchangeably.
2. Work (W): A force moving through a distance ($W = F \times d$, where d = distance). Typical units of work are kp·m, kg·m, ft·lbs, N·m, and joules (J)*. The metabolic equivalent of work is the total energy expended (E) in performing the mechanical work. A typical unit of E is kcals (Calories).
3. Power (P): The rate at which work is being done ($P = W \cdot t^{-1}$‡ where t = time). Typical units of power are $kp \cdot m \cdot min^{-1}$, $kg \cdot m \cdot min^{-1}$, $J \cdot min^{-1}$ and watts (W)*. The metabolic equivalent of power is the rate of energy expenditure ($\dot{E}$) that occurs in response to the imposed mechanical work rate or power. Typical units of $\dot{E}$ are METs and $\dot{V}O_2$. It is $\dot{E}$ with which we are most concerned clinically. Non-weight bearing activities (e.g. cycle ergometry) are measured in units of absolute power. Measures of *absolute* mechanical power include $kp \cdot m \cdot min^{-1}$, $kg \cdot m \cdot min^{-1}$ and watts*. *Absolute* measures of $\dot{E}$ are $kcal \cdot min^{-1}$, $l\ O_2 \cdot min^{-1}$ and $ml\ O_2 \cdot min^{-1}$. Weight bearing activities (e.g. jogging) are measured in units of relative power. *Relative* measures of $\dot{E}$ include METs and $ml\ O_2 \cdot$(kg body

*Preferred SI unit.

‡Please note: The notation $W \cdot t^{-1}$ is equivalent to W/t i.e. the superscript "$^{-1}$" can be read as "divided by" or "per" as in work divided by time or work per unit time.

weight)$^{-1}\cdot$min^{-1}, which is usually written ml·kg$^{-1}\cdot$min^{-1}. Note that relative measures of $\dot{E}$ are all expressed "per kg body weight".

4. METs: A multiple of the resting rate of O_2 consumption ($\dot{V}O_{2rest}$). One MET equals $\dot{V}O_{2rest}$ which is approximately 3.5 ml·kg$^{-1}\cdot$min^{-1}; it represents the approximate rate of O_2 consumption of a seated individual at rest. Thus, an individual exercising at 2 METs is consuming O_2 at twice the resting rate (i.e., 7 ml·kg$^{-1}\cdot$min^{-1}), while an individual exercising at 10 METs is consuming O_2 at 10 times the resting rate (i.e., 35 ml·kg$^{-1}\cdot$min^{-1}).

Conversions and Useful Relationships

Distance:
 1 mi = 1.6 km*
Speed:
 1 mi·h^{-1} = 26.8 m·min^{-1}
Weight:
 1 kg = 1 kp = 9.8 N*
 1 kg = 2.2 lb
Work:
 1 kcal = 4.2 kJ*
 1 l O_2 ≅ 5 kcal
 1 kg·m ≅ 1.8 ml O_2
Power:
 1 watt* = 1 J·s^{-1} = 1 N·m·sec^{-1}
 1 watt* = 6.1 kg·m·min^{-1} ≅ 6.0 kg·m·min^{-1}
 1 MET = 3.5 ml·kg$^{-1}\cdot$min^{-1}
 1 MET ≅ 1 kcal·kg$^{-1}\cdot$h^{-1}
 1 MET ≅ 1.6 km·h^{-1}†
 1 MET ≅ 1.0 mi·h^{-1}†

*SI units
†for running on a horizontal surface

Usage

Table D–1 summarizes the important steps in calculating the rate of whole body work for a variety of standard activities. Note that for each activity, there are three components of $\dot{E}$ to be considered: horizontal, vertical or resistive, and resting. Summing these individual components gives the total $\dot{E}$ output during that activity. These equations can be used to estimate steady state $\dot{E}$ as well as to calculate what combination of speed/grade or weight/rpm applied to the mode will yield a desired $\dot{E}$. The calculations are done in units of $\dot{V}O_2$ ($ml \cdot kg^{-1} \cdot min^{-1}$ or $ml \cdot min^{-1}$). It is easiest to perform all calculations in these units and then convert to METs, SI units, or other units as appropriate for your final answer.

Cautions

Direct determination of oxygen consumption is the standard measure of the metabolic response to exercise. This measurement requires the use of a breathing valve for collection and analysis of expired air during exercise. The $\dot{V}O_2$ for a given level of exercise is highly reproducible in a given individual; however, studies indicate that the measured $\dot{V}O_2$ at any given running speed, walking speed/grade will vary between individuals by approximately 7%. $\dot{V}O_2$ for a given activity is relatively unaffected by the environment, except in the presence of factors that may alter the mechanical work of the activity such as wind, snow or sand.

Due to the difficulty in direct measurement of $\dot{V}O_2$, equations have been derived to estimate the metabolic equivalent of a given activity. This estimate of the $\dot{V}O_2$ (or METs) is valid primarily for steady state exercise. When used to determine the metabolic equivalent of non-steady state or maximal workrate, it must be recognized that the measured $\dot{V}O_2$ may differ from estimated for two reasons: 1) if a steady state is not yet reached, the measured $\dot{V}O_2$ is less than the estimated $\dot{V}O_2$ and 2) exercise at maximal and near maximal intensities involves both aerobic and anaerobic components, which will result in an over-estimated MET level due to the unknown contribution of the anaerobic component to the exercise. The use of these equations to estimate METs, despite the discussed problems, is typically used in clinical settings to indicate the metabolic response to exercise on a treadmill or cycle ergometer. These formulae only give estimates of $\dot{V}O_2$ or METs.

Estimated METs can be used as a guideline for exercise prescription of activities in a neutral environment. The metabolic response to a given exercise (e.g. jogging at 161 $m \cdot min^{-1}$) against a wind (which increases the external work which must be performed) is higher than the same exercise performed on the treadmill in a neutral environment. The use of METs for activity prescription should, therefore, be used carefully. Subjects should know appropriate heart rates for the activity and should check their heart rate response regularly. This is especially important in patients with ischemic heart disease, since approximately 80% of the increase in myocardial oxygen demand with exercise in the non-failing heart is a result of the increase in heart rate. Thus, heart rate is a much better indicator than estimated MET level of the appropriate exercise intensity relative to the myocardial oxygen supply/demand status.

Estimation of METs is also advantageous in exercise testing to express the metabolic response to external work. This provides a way to compare various treadmill protocols which use various combinations of speed and grade. Evaluation of progress in an exercise program can also be assessed in the same individual using estimated max METs, bearing in mind the limitation of estimation of max $\dot{V}O_2$ outlined above. Finally, without properly calibrated equipment, or with rail-holding during treadmill exercise, calculated $\dot{V}O_2$'s or METs are inaccurate and unreliable.

Walking

$\dot{V}O_2$ can be estimated with reasonable accuracy for walking speeds from 50 to 100 $m \cdot min^{-1}$ (1.9 to 3.7 $mi \cdot h^{-1}$). The O_2 cost of horizontal walking is 0.1 $ml \cdot kg^{-1} \cdot min^{-1}$ per $m \cdot min^{-1}$ of horizontal velocity $\left(\frac{0.1\ ml \cdot kg^{-1} \cdot min^{-1}}{m \cdot min^{-1}}\right)$. The O_2 cost of vertical work is $1.8\ ml \cdot kg^{-1} \cdot m^{-1} = \left(\frac{1.8\ ml \cdot kg^{-1} \cdot min^{-1}}{m \cdot min^{-1}}\right)$. (See Table D–1, walking, comment #2.) Since we do not walk up a vertical treadmill, the component of vertical work done is estimated by multiplying the O_2 cost of vertical work by treadmill grade (as a fraction) and speed. The resting component is one MET which equals 3.5 $ml \cdot kg^{-1} \cdot min^{-1}$.

Although $\dot{V}O_2$ estimates for walking are relatively accurate for most speeds and grades, there are exceptions. For example, the formula is more accurate in estimating $\dot{V}O_2$ when the participant is walking up a grade than on the level. Underestimates of 15 to 20% are expected with level walking, and 5 to 8% with walking up a 3% grade. Also, children are less efficient in walking and running than adults. The walking formula underestimates the oxygen requirement by approximately 0.5

$ml \cdot kg^{-1} \cdot min^{-1}$ for each year of age below the age of 18 years. The walking formula is equally accurate for men and women across the adult age range.

Running/Jogging

$\dot{V}O_2$ can be estimated with reasonable accuracy for speeds in excess of 134 $m \cdot min^{-1}$ (5 $mi \cdot h^{-1}$) and even for speeds as low as 80 $m \cdot min^{-1}$ (3 $mi \cdot h^{-1}$) if the subject is truly jogging (not walking). The O_2 cost of horizontal running at a given speed is about twice that for walking since running generally is a less efficient process than walking at lower speeds. High speed walking (>134 $m \cdot min^{-1}$) is also less efficient than running at the same speed. The vertical component of running on the treadmill is different from treadmill walking. When running up small grades some of the vertical lift normally found in level running is used to accomplish grade work, reducing the O_2 cost of grade work. This can be effectively corrected by multiplying the vertical component of the treadmill running by 0.5. Again, the resting component must be included. Since the O_2 cost of grade running off the treadmill may not be reliably predicted, the equation does not apply to this activity.

Leg Ergometry

$\dot{V}O_2$ can be estimated with reasonable accuracy for work rates between 300 to 1200 $kg \cdot m \cdot min^{-1}$ (50 to 200 watts*). There is no horizontal component to cycle ergometry since the cycle is stationary. Except in the cases of extremely obese or slight individuals, the mechanical work rate or power of cycling is related to the set resistance and revolutions per min and is independent of body weight. Thus, a given person weighing 60 kg will have the same absolute $\dot{V}O_2$ (i.e., in $ml \cdot min^{-1}$) at a given mechanical power on the cycle ergometer as a person weighing 90 kg. However, if expressed relative to body weight (i.e., in METs or $ml \cdot kg^{-1} \cdot min^{-1}$), the lighter individual would have a greater relative $\dot{V}O_2$. The mechanical power (in $kg \cdot m \cdot min^{-1}$) is determined by the product of the weight applied (kg or kp), the distance this weight travels per revolution ($m \cdot rev^{-1}$) and the number of revolutions per minute ($rev \cdot min^{-1}$), or $kg \cdot m \cdot min^{-1} = (kg) \times (m \cdot rev^{-1}) \times (rev \cdot min^{-1})$. This power term should ultimately be converted into SI units by using the relationship 1 W = 6 $kg \cdot m \cdot min^{-1}$. It should be noted that two common ergometers, the Monarch and the Tunturi, travel 6 $m \cdot rev^{-1}$ and

3 m·rev^{-1}, respectively. To fully account for the added frictional work in the ergometer, the O_2 cost of the vertical or resistive work (1.8 ml·kg^{-1}·m^{-1}) is augmented by 0.2 ml·kg^{-1}·m^{-1} so that for cycle ergometry the O_2 cost of work against the applied load equals the sum of these two values or 2.0 ml·kg^{-1}·m^{-1}. The resting component of O_2 consumption (corrected for body weight) is again added to obtain the total $\dot{V}O_2$.

Arm Ergometry

$\dot{V}O_2$ can be estimated with reasonable accuracy for work rates between 150 and 750 kg·m·min^{-1} (25 to 125 watts*). The same considerations that apply to leg ergometry apply to arm ergometry; however, different constants apply. The O_2 cost of the resistive component (3.0 ml·kg^{-1}·min^{-1}) is larger than seen with other modes. This is most likely due to the involvement of considerable accessory musculature to stabilize the upper body during arm ergometry. The resting component of oxygen consumption corrected for body weight is again added to obtain the total $\dot{V}O_2$. Since the relationship between a person's $\dot{V}O_{2max}$ with leg ergometry and arm ergometry may be weak, it is important to do arm ergometry on individuals whose major occupational or leisure activities involve arm vs leg work. Furthermore, since the heart rate response to arm ergometry exceeds that seen at the same submaximal work rate in leg ergometry and since peak heart rate is less in arm than leg ergometry, arm ergometry testing is important for exercise prescription where arm work comprises a substantial portion of the exercise program.

Stepping

$\dot{V}O_2$ of bench and stair stepping varies with stepping rate, step height, and whether the person is stepping up or down or both. The O_2 cost of the horizontal component of stepping equals about 0.35 ml·kg^{-1}·min^{-1} per steps·min^{-1} or $0.35\left(\frac{\text{ml·kg}^{-1}\text{·min}^{-1}}{\text{steps·min}^{-1}}\right)$. The O_2 cost of the vertical component of stepping depends upon the stepping rate (steps·min^{-1}), the step height (m·step^{-1}), and whether the person is stepping up, down, or both. The O_2 cost of stepping down is about 1/3 that of stepping up so for each complete cycle (up and down) the

O_2 cost is 1.33 times the O_2 cost of stepping up alone. Since the O_2 cost of vertical work is $\frac{1.8\ ml \cdot kg^{-1} \cdot min^{-1}}{m \cdot min^{-1}}$, the vertical O_2 cost for up and down stepping is $(m \cdot steps^{-1}) \times (steps \cdot min^{-1}) \times 1.33 \times \left(\frac{1.8\ ml \cdot kg^{-1} \cdot min^{-1}}{m \cdot min^{-1}}\right)$. Note that stepping height must be in meters, not centimeter or inches. The resting component has been included in the horizontal and vertical components.

Miscellaneous Activities

Rope skipping is convenient and requires the expenditure of a large number of calories, but it is difficult to vary the intensity of work and may be inappropriate for the average sedentary American or the typical patient with ischemic heart disease. Skipping at 60 to 80 skips·min^{-1} requires approximately nine METs. Doubling the rate of skipping to 120 to 140 skips·min^{-1} increases the work rate to 11 to 12 METs. Furthermore, the heart rate response tends to be higher than expected at comparable MET levels for walking or running. Thus, even the lowest rate of skipping (60–80 skips·min^{-1}) requires a MET level close to the maximum METs of the typical sedentary adult. In addition, this high MET level and the exaggerated heart rate response would tend to preclude rope skipping as an activity by the average patient with ischemic heart disease.

It is also difficult to vary the intensity of effort during rebound running on a mini-trampoline, since stepping rate varies little while an individual maintains a "normal" rebound height. Rebound running at the average stepping rate of 60 steps·min^{-1} requires approximately five METs. Due to the low acceleration forces seen with this activity, it may be a recommended activity for those individuals with lower extremity injuries who require moderate rates of energy expenditure. Exercise heart rate is not a good estimate of exercise intensity during rebound running.

Swimming is another activity which is difficult to grade due to the large differences in stroke efficiency among individuals. Average heart rates at a given submaximal $\dot{V}O_2$ are about 20 b·min^{-1} lower (range 5–50 b·min^{-1}) in the water than on land for walking activities requiring the same $\dot{V}O_2$. This decreases myocardial oxygen demand; however, maximal heart rates may also be lower in the water. Thus, a training heart rate based on a treadmill test may be too high during swimming activities and may need to be reduced to protect against early fatigue.

The energy cost of outdoor bicycling is also difficult to predict because it varies with bicycle characteristics, speed, grade and wind resistance. Wind resistance is related to frontal surface area of the cyclist which is a function of body weight. Therefore, the absolute oxygen cost of cycling in the ambient environment will be greater for the heavier individual than for the lighter one, all other conditions being similar. This is different from what is seen in laboratory cycle ergometry where individuals of different weights will have similar rates of oxygen consumption under similar experimental conditions.

The energy cost of aerobic dancing is also difficult to quantitate. Low intensity dancing (e.g., walking through the routine without overhead hand motion) requires about 3.5 METs while medium intensity dancing requires about five METs and high intensity dancing requires about nine METs.

Calculations

Table D–1 gives a visual presentation of how metabolic calculations may be done. The table is intended to be used as a guide for calculating various components of the energy cost formulas. The examples that follow show how various components of the energy cost formulae can be calculated. Always pay attention to units. Always place the appropriate units next to each quantity. If your units do not cancel to give the appropriate units for your answers, either your approach or your answer is incorrect.

Example 1:

Calculate the $\dot{E}$ in units of $ml \cdot kg^{-1} \cdot min^{-1}$ ($\dot{V}O_2$) and METs of the following activity:

treadmill speed = $2.5\ mi \cdot h^{-1}$
treadmill grade = 12 %
subject weight = 175 pounds

a) convert speed to $m \cdot min^{-1}$; note that subject weight does not enter into this calculation

$$(2.5\ \not{mi} \cdot \not{h}^{-1}) \times \left(\frac{26.8\ m \cdot min^{-1}}{\not{mi} \cdot \not{h}^{-1}}\right) = 67\ m \cdot min^{-1}$$

(Note that the slashes indicate cancellation of units.)

b) calculate horizontal component (HC)

$$HC = (m \cdot min^{-1}) \times \left(\frac{0.1\ ml \cdot kg^{-1} \cdot min^{-1}}{m \cdot min^{-1}}\right)$$

$$= (67\ \not{m} \cdot \not{min}^{-1}) \times \left(\frac{0.1\ ml \cdot kg^{-1} \cdot min^{-1}}{\not{m} \cdot \not{min}^{-1}}\right)$$

$$= 6.7\ ml \cdot kg^{-1} \cdot min^{-1}$$

c) calculate vertical component (VC); note that grade must be a fraction

$$VC = (grade) \times (m \cdot min^{-1}) \times \left(\frac{1.8\ ml \cdot kg^{-1} \cdot min^{-1}}{m \cdot min^{-1}}\right)$$

$$= (.12) \times (67\ \not{m} \cdot \not{min}^{-1}) \times \left(\frac{1.8\ ml \cdot kg^{-1} \cdot min^{-1}}{\not{m} \cdot \not{min}^{-1}}\right)$$

$$= 14.5\ ml \cdot kg^{-1} \cdot min^{-1}$$

d) calculate $\dot{V}O_2$ in $ml \cdot kg^{-1} \cdot min^{-1}$

$\dot{V}O_2 = (HC) + (VC) + Rest$

$= (6.7\ ml \cdot kg^{-1} \cdot min^{-1}) + (14.5\ ml \cdot kg^{-1} \cdot min^{-1}) + (3.5\ ml \cdot kg^{-1} \cdot min^{-1})$

$= 24.7\ ml \cdot kg^{-1} \cdot min^{-1}$

e) calculate $\dot{E}$ in METs by converting $\dot{V}O_2$ to METs

$$\dot{E} = \dot{V}O_2 \times \left(\frac{1\ MET}{3.5\ ml \cdot kg^{-1} \cdot min^{-1}}\right)$$

$$= (24.7\ \not{ml} \cdot \not{kg}^{-1} \cdot \not{min}^{-1}) \times \left(\frac{1\ MET}{3.5\ \not{ml} \cdot \not{kg}^{-1} \cdot \not{min}^{-1}}\right)$$

$$= 7.1\ METs$$

Example 2

A subject has a maximal exercise capacity of 12 METs. The exercise prescription is for 70% of maximal capacity using a cycle ergometer. Calculate the mechanical power appropriate to obtain this prescribed level. The subject weighs 172 lbs. Note: Our approach is to solve for the mechanical power term $\left(\frac{kg \cdot m}{min}\right)$ in the resistive component and convert to SI units. For clarity of illustration, this calculation has been split into its component parts.

a) convert lbs to kgs

$$(172\ \text{lb}) \times \left(\frac{1\ \text{kg}}{2.2\ \text{lbs}}\right) = 78.2\ \text{kg}$$

b) calculate training METs

$$\begin{aligned}\dot{E} &= 0.70 \times \dot{E}_{max} \\ &= (0.70) \times 12\ \text{METs} \\ &= 8.4\ \text{METs}\end{aligned}$$

c) calculate training $\dot{V}O_2$ (in $ml \cdot kg^{-1} \cdot min^{-1}$)

$$\begin{aligned}\dot{V}O_2 &= \dot{E}\ (\text{METs}) \times \left(\frac{3.5\ ml \cdot kg^{-1} \cdot min^{-1}}{1\ \text{MET}}\right) \\ &= (8.4\ \text{METs}) \times \left(\frac{3.5\ ml \cdot kg^{-1} \cdot min^{-1}}{1\ \text{MET}}\right) \\ &= 29.4\ ml \cdot kg^{-1} \cdot min^{-1}\end{aligned}$$

d) convert relative $\dot{V}O_2$ to absolute $\dot{V}O_2$

$$\begin{aligned}\dot{V}O_2\ (ml \cdot min^{-1}) &= \dot{V}O_2\ (ml \cdot kg^{-1} \cdot min^{-1}) \times \text{Body weight (kg)} \\ &= (29.4\ ml \cdot kg^{-1} \cdot min^{-1}) \times (78.2\ kg) \\ &= 2299\ ml \cdot min^{-1}\end{aligned}$$

e) calculate resting component (Rest)

$$\begin{aligned}\text{Rest} &= 3.5\ ml \cdot kg^{-1} \cdot min^{-1} \times kg\ \text{(body weight)} \\ &= 3.5\ ml \cdot kg^{-1} \cdot min^{-1} \times 78.2\ kg \\ &= 274\ ml \cdot min^{-1}\end{aligned}$$

f) use leg ergometry formula to calculate the resistive component (RC)

$$\begin{aligned}\dot{V}O_2 &= HC + RC + \text{Rest} \\ &= O + RC + \text{Rest} \\ &= RC + \text{Rest}\end{aligned}$$

$$\begin{aligned}\therefore RC &= \dot{V}O_2 - \text{Rest} \\ &= 2299\ ml \cdot min^{-1} - 274\ ml \cdot min^{-1} \\ &= 2025\ ml \cdot min^{-1}\end{aligned}$$

g) calculate mechanical power (P) from RC

$$RC\ (ml \cdot min^{-1}) = P\ (kg \cdot m \cdot min^{-1}) \times 2\ (ml \cdot kg^{-1} \cdot m^{-1})$$

$$\begin{aligned}\therefore P &= \frac{RC\ (ml \cdot min^{-1})}{2\ (ml \cdot kg^{-1} \cdot m^{-1})} \\ &= \frac{2025\ ml \cdot min^{-1}}{2\ ml \cdot kg^{-1} \cdot m^{-1}} \\ &= 1013\ kg \cdot m \cdot min^{-1}\end{aligned}$$

Table D-1. Summary of Metabolic Calculations

$\dot{V}O_2$ Mode (units)	=	Horizontal Components	+	Vertical or Resistive Component	+	Resting Component	Comments
Walking $(ml \cdot kg^{-1} \cdot min^{-1})$	=	$m \cdot min^{-1} \times \left(0.1 \frac{ml \cdot kg^{-1} \cdot min^{-1}}{m \cdot min^{-1}}\right)$	+	grade (frac) × $m \cdot min^{-1} \times 1.8 \frac{ml \cdot kg^{-1} \cdot min^{-1}}{m \cdot min^{-1}}$	+	$3.5\ ml \cdot kg^{-1} \cdot min^{-1}$	1. For speeds of 50–100 $m \cdot min^{-1}$ (1.9–3.7 $mi \cdot h^{-1}$) 2. $1.8 \frac{ml}{kg \cdot m} \times \frac{m \cdot min^{-1}}{m \cdot min^{-1}} = 1.8 \frac{ml \cdot kg^{-1} \cdot min^{-1}}{m \cdot min^{-1}}$ 3. 1 $mi \cdot h^{-1}$ = 26.8 $m \cdot min^{-1}$
Running $(ml \cdot kg^{-1} \cdot min^{-1})$	=	$m \cdot min^{-1} \times \left(0.2 \frac{ml \cdot kg^{-1} \cdot min^{-1}}{m \cdot min^{-1}}\right)$ ▲	+	grade (frac) × $m \cdot min^{-1} \times 1.8 \frac{ml \cdot kg^{-1} \cdot min^{-1}}{m \cdot min^{-1}} \times 0.5$ ▲	+	$3.5\ ml \cdot kg^{-1} \cdot min^{-1}$	1. For speeds >134 $m \cdot min^{-1}$ (>5.0 $mi \cdot h^{-1}$) 2. If truly jogging (not walking), this equation can also be used for speeds between 80 and 134 $m \cdot min^{-1}$ (3–5 $mi \cdot h^{-1}$) 3. Formula applies to level running off the treadmill, but not to grade running off the treadmill
Leg Ergometer $(ml \cdot min^{-1})$	=	None	+	$\frac{kg \cdot m}{min} \times \frac{2\ ml}{kg \cdot m}$	+	$3.5\ ml \cdot kg^{-1} \cdot min^{-1} \times$ kg (BW)	1. For work rates between 300–1200 $kg \cdot m \cdot min^{-1}$ 2. $\frac{kg \cdot m}{min} = kg \times \frac{m}{rev} \times \frac{rev}{min}$

				▲		▲	3. Multiply resting component by body weight (kg) to convert to $ml \cdot min^{-1}$ 4. Monarch = $6\ m \cdot rev^{-1}$ Tunturi = $3\ m \cdot rev^{-1}$
▨ Arm Ergometer ($ml \cdot min^{-1}$)	+	None	+	▨ $\frac{kg \cdot m}{min} \times 3 \frac{ml}{kg \cdot m}$ ▲	+	$3.5\ ml \cdot kg^{-1} \cdot min^{-1} \times kg$ (BW) ▲	1. For work rates between 150–750 $kg \cdot m \cdot min^{-1}$ 2. $\frac{kg \cdot m}{min} = kg \times \frac{m}{rev} \times \frac{rev}{min}$ 3. Multiply resting component by body weight (kg) to convert to $ml \cdot min^{-1}$
▨ Stepping ($ml \cdot kg^{-1} \cdot min^{-1}$)	=	▨ $\frac{steps}{min} \times 0.35 \frac{ml \cdot kg^{-1} \cdot min^{-1}}{steps \cdot min^{-1}}$ ▲	+	▨ ▨ $\frac{m}{steps} \times \frac{steps}{min} \times 1.33 \times 1.8 \frac{ml \cdot kg^{-1} \cdot min^{-1}}{m \cdot min^{-1}}$	+	Included in horizontal and vertical components ▲	1. 1.33 includes both positive component of going up (1.0) + negative component of going down (0.33) = 1.33 2. Stepping height in meters.

Key: ▨ possible unknown quantity
▲ note change in constant

h) convert kg·m·min^{-1} to watts, the appropriate SI unit

$$P\ (\text{watts}) = P\ (\text{kg·m·min}^{-1}) \times \left(\frac{1\ \text{watt}}{6\ \text{kg·m·min}^{-1}}\right)$$

$$= (1013\ \text{kg·m·min}^{-1}) \times \left(\frac{1\ \text{watt}}{6\ \text{kg·m·min}^{-1}}\right)$$

$$= 169\ \text{watts}$$

Example 3:

If the subject in example 2 desired to pedal at 80 rpm (rev·min^{-1}) on an ergometer with a flywheel that travels 6 m·rev^{-1}, how much weight or load should be placed on the ergometer?

a) calculate weight or force (F) applied in kg

$$P\ (\text{kg·m·min}^{-1}) = F\ (\text{kg}) \times (\text{m·rev}^{-1}) \times (\text{rev·min}^{-1})$$

$$\therefore F\ (\text{kg}) = \frac{P\ (\text{kg·m·min}^{-1})}{(\text{m·rev}^{-1}) \times (\text{rev·min}^{-1})}$$

$$= \frac{1013\ \text{kg·m·min}^{-1}}{(6\ \text{m·rev}^{-1}) \times (80\ \text{rev·min}^{-1})}$$

$$= 2.1\ \text{kg}$$

Table D–2. Approximate Energy Requirements in METs For Horizontal and Grade Walking

% Grade	*mi·h^{-1}*	*1.7*	*2.0*	*2.5*	*3.0*	*3.4*	*3.75*
	m·min^{-1}	*45.6*	*53.7*	*67.0*	*80.5*	*91.2*	*100.5*
0		2.3	2.5	2.9	3.3	3.6	3.9
2.5		2.9	3.2	3.8	4.3	4.8	5.2
5.0		3.5	3.9	4.6	5.4	5.9	6.5
7.5		4.1	4.6	5.5	6.4	7.1	7.8
10.0		4.6	5.3	6.3	7.4	8.3	9.1
12.5		5.2	6.0	7.2	8.5	9.5	10.4
15.0		5.8	6.6	8.1	9.5	10.6	11.7
17.5		6.4	7.3	8.9	10.5	11.8	12.9
20.0		7.0	8.0	9.8	11.6	13.0	14.2
22.5		7.6	8.7	10.6	12.6	14.2	15.5
25.0		8.2	9.4	11.5	13.6	15.3	16.8

Table D-3. Approximate Energy Requirements in METS for Horizontal and Uphill Jogging/Running

a. Outdoors on solid surface

% Grade	$m \cdot h^{-1}$	5	6	7	7.5	8	9	10
	$m \cdot min^{-1}$	134	161	188	201	215	241	268
0		8.6	10.2	11.7	12.5	13.3	14.8	16.3
2.5		10.3	12.3	14.1	15.1	16.1	17.9	19.7
5.0		12.0	14.3	16.5	17.7	18.8		
7.5		13.8	16.4	18.9				
10.0		15.5	18.5					

b. On the treadmill

% Grade	$m \cdot h^{-1}$	5	6	7	7.5	8	9	10
	$m \cdot min^{-1}$	134	161	188	201	215	241	268
0		8.6	10.2	11.7	12.5	13.3	14.8	16.3
2.5		9.5	11.2	12.9	13.8	14.7	16.3	18.0
5.0		10.3	12.3	14.1	15.1	16.1	17.9	19.7
7.5		11.2	13.3	15.3	16.4	17.4	19.4	
10.0		12.0	14.3	16.5	17.7	18.8		
12.5		12.9	15.4	17.7	19.0			
15.0		13.8	16.4	18.9				

Table D–4. Approximate Energy Expenditure in METs During Bicycle Ergometry

Body Weight		*Exercise Rate ($kg \cdot m \cdot min^{-1}$ and Watts)*						
kg	*lbs*	*300* *50*	*450* *75*	*600* *100*	*750* *125*	*900* *150*	*1050* *175*	*1200 ($kg \cdot m \cdot min^{-1}$),* *200 (Watts)*
50	110	5.1	6.9	8.6	10.3	12.0	13.7	15.4
60	132	4.3	5.7	7.1	8.6	10.0	11.4	12.9
70	154	3.7	4.9	6.1	7.3	8.6	9.8	11.0
80	176	3.2	4.3	5.4	6.4	7.5	8.6	9.6
90	198	2.9	3.8	4.8	5.7	6.7	7.6	8.6
100	220	2.6	3.4	4.3	5.1	6.0	6.9	7.7

NOTE: $\dot{V}O_2$ for zero load pedaling is approximately 550 $ml \cdot min^{-1}$ for 70 to 80 kg subjects.

SELECTED REFERENCES

Adams, WC: Influence of age, sex and body weight on the energy expenditure of bicycle riding. *J. Appl. Physiol. 22*:539–545, 1967.

Astrand, PO: Work tests with the bicycle ergometer. Varberg, Sweden: Monark-Crescent AB, (undated).

Claremont, A, Reddan WG, Smith, EL: Metabolic costs and feasibility of water support exercises for the elderly. In: Nagle FJ, Montoye HJ, (eds). *Exercise in Health and Disease.* Springfield: Charles C Thomas, 1981, pp. 215–225.

Dill, DB: Oxygen used in horizontal and grade walking and running on the treadmill. *J. Appl. Physiol. 20*:19–22, 1965.

Franklin BA, Vander L, Wrisley D, Rubenfire M: Aerobic requirements of arm ergometry: implications for exercise testing and training. *Phys. Spts. Med. 11*:81–90, 1983.

Katch VL, Villanacci JF, and Sady, SP: Energy costs of rebound-running. *Res. Quart. Exer. Spt. 52*:269–272, 1981.

Knuttgen, HG: Force, work, power and exercise. *Med. Sci. Spts. 10*:227–228, 1978.

Legwold G: Does aerobic dance offer more fun than fitness? *Phys. Spts. Med. 10*:147–151, 1982.

Magaria R, et al: Energy cost of running. *J. Appl. Physiol. 18*:367–370, 1963.

Nagle FJ, Balke B, and Naughton JP: Gradational step tests for assessing work capacity. *J. Appl. Physiol. 20*:745–748, 1965.

Nagle FJ, et al: Compatability of progressive treadmill, bicycle and step tests based on oxygen uptake responses. *Med. Sci. Spts. 3*:149–154, 1971.

Passmore R, Durnin JVGA: Human energy expenditure. *Physiol. Rev. 35*:801–840, 1955.

Index

Page numbers followed by "t" refer to tables. Page numbers in *italics* indicate figures.